Si King & Dave Myers

THE HAIRY
DIETERS

EAT FOR LIFE

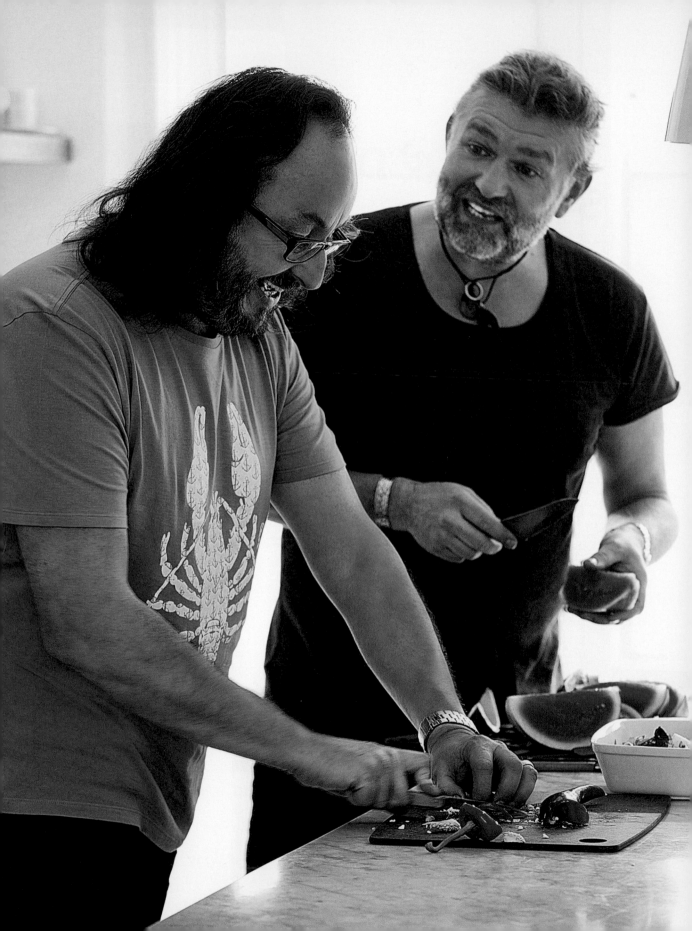

Si King & Dave Myers

THE HAIRY DIETERS

EAT FOR LIFE

with Justine Pattison

WEIDENFELD & NICOLSON

We'd like to dedicate this book to all the lovely people who've bought the book, got on the scales and are giving the diet a go – more power to your elbow and waistline. Love and good luck,

Si & Dave x

First published in Great Britain in 2013 by
Weidenfeld & Nicolson, an imprint of the Orion Publishing Group Ltd
Orion House, 5 Upper St Martin's Lane, London WC2H 9EA
An Hachette UK Company

10 9 8 7 6 5

A CIP catalogue record for this book is available from the British Library.

ISBN: 978 0 297 87047 0

Photographer: Andrew Hayes-Watkins
Food stylists: Lisa Harrison and Anna Burges-Lumsden
Designer and prop stylist: Loulou Clark
Editor: Jinny Johnson
Proofreader: Elise See Tai
Indexer: Elizabeth Wiggans
Food styling assistants: Victoria Grier, Alice Porter
Photographer's assistant: Kristy Noble

Nutritional analysis calculated by:
Lauren Brignell (BSc Hons Nutrition)

Printed and bound in Germany by Mohn Media

optomen

CONTENTS

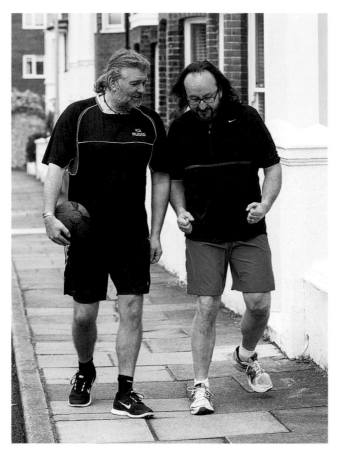

Never in our wildest dreams did we think that our battles with our weight would strike so many chords with so many people. We've been overwhelmed by the response to our first *Hairy Dieters* book and thrilled that you've all found it as useful as we have. We love the way everyone is sharing the pain – and more importantly the gains – and we feel there's now a great community of Hairy Dieters out there!

As most of you now know, the reason we started this diet was simple: we had got really big. We were morbidly obese. There, we've said it. We were fat, we were on tablets, we felt rough. But food was our life, our career, our passion and our comfort – how could we think of dieting? Fortunately we got our act together before it was too late and we discovered we didn't need to lose our enthusiasm for food. In fact, we love it more than ever. Who would have thought it would be such fun to experiment with recipes that pile on the flavour without the pounds?

We had to work hard at it for a few months but we achieved our goals. A year on, we're pleased to say that we've kept the weight off and this way of eating has become a way of life. We've changed how we cook and how we think about food and recipes. And we think we're better cooks because of it. We find there is a cleanness and freshness to our food now and we're more creative with textures and tastes. Our mantra is that first and foremost our diet recipes are great food. It just so happens that they have the wonderful bonus of being less calorific.

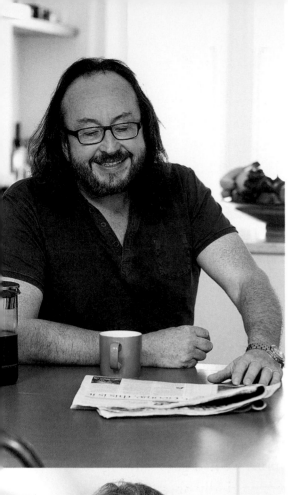

BIKERS LITE

To be honest, at one stage, we weren't sure we'd be able to stick with the diet, but the idea of being weighed before millions of viewers every week sure does pile on the pressure. We couldn't have coped with the shame if those scales hadn't started to drop. And thank goodness that our great recipes made it all a lot easier than we'd thought.

What we didn't realise would happen, and what has kept us going, is how much better we feel. Our blood pressure is down, our cholesterol levels are healthy and we've more energy than we had 10 years ago. We're better tempered, our families say, and nicer to live with.

What's more, it's so great to walk into a clothes shop and not to have to head for the fat boy rail. We've bought skinny jeans and posh trousers straight off the peg and it feels fantastic. Makes it all the easier to keep ourselves on the straight and calorie-controlled narrrow.

TAKING CONTROL

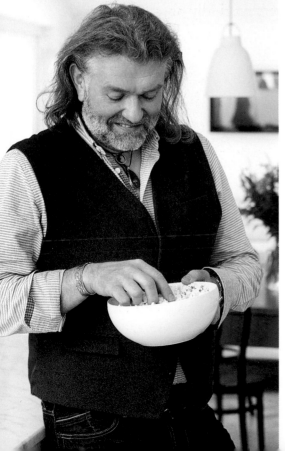

We're never going to be skinny but we have shed a lot of weight and now we're not sticking to a strict 1,500 calories a day or whatever week after week for ever. That wouldn't be healthy. But we do try to make sure we don't overeat and we've got into the habit of cooking with less fat, watching the carbs and not piling our plates too high. Of course, there have been times when we've fallen off the wagon – Christmas, birthday weekends, the occasional craving for fast food. There was a day recently when we gave in to a major burger craving round the back of a service station! Happens to us all but you know what? It didn't taste that great.

What we've discovered is that if one day you overdo it a bit and have a blowout lunch or too much cake, don't beat yourself up about it. Enjoy the treat and just be extra careful the next day or so. We're not frightened to get on the scales now and we both weigh ourselves every week.

We're lucky that we've been able to make this journey together and we've been able to support each other. We know that many of you are shedding the pounds with a partner or buddy and loads of people have found support in our online diet club. It does make a difference if you have someone to encourage you when you're feeling like it's all too much.

We feel we've taken control of our lives and ourselves and that's vital for our self-respect. We've found a sustainable way of life as far as our food is concerned and if we have the odd little naughty moment here and there – well, we can cope.

A BOOKFUL OF NEW RECIPES

We've cooked the recipes in our first book over and over, and they've become much-loved standards in our kitchens, along with our other favourite dishes. We enjoy them so much that, like you, we wanted more, so over the last year we've come up with some new ones that we hope you're going to like just as much. As before, these are lower-calorie recipes to help you lose weight in a calorie-controlled diet. And again, what we love about them is that they taste like real food, not diet food, and you can make them every night of the week. They've got that satisfying, great-in-your-mouth feeling that lets you know you've eaten something. You can eat entirely from the book or use it some of the time to maintain your weight loss – or to drop the odd pound when you've been overdoing it. Like the other recipes, these are good for the whole family – just up the side dishes for the stringbeans among you and they'll never know the difference.

As we've been developing these new recipes we've been thinking a lot about tricks and techniques that help to keep the calorie count down without losing flavour; little things like trimming the fat off your meat and brushing or spraying a pan with oil instead of pouring it in like we always used to do. We eat far more veg now than before and we love our salads. And we've really cut down on the sugar.

A FEW POINTERS FROM US

A calorie is a unit of energy contained in food. We burn calories for energy, but if we take in more than we need, they're stored as fat. We've given calorie counts for all our recipes so you can keep yourself in line. On some packages you'll see the term kilocalories, but this is just the proper name for calories – they're the same thing. You might also see a figure in kilojoules – another way of measuring food energy – but don't worry about these.

Now, we know you're not greedy like us, but don't be tempted to eat more than your fair share of these recipes. Most are for two or four people so don't think you can scoff the lot and still drop the weight.

We always weigh everything carefully and use proper spoons and a measuring jug. Otherwise you'll change the calorie count. Makes sense doesn't it? You'll notice we often mention spray oil (try to buy the most natural kind) but if you prefer, just brush on a small amount of oil.

You'll notice that we list small amounts of some high-cal ingredients such as Parmesan cheese. Don't worry, it's fine. The taste of these things is so good and strong you don't need much to flavour your dish. Onions and garlic should be peeled unless otherwise specified. And we like to use free-range eggs and chicken whenever possible.

Si: For me, cutting back on the booze has been the hardest bit. Trouble is that not only does alcohol have loads of calories, it also weakens your willpower so once you've had one drink it's all too easy to have another, and another. Then the demon gets into you and before you know it you're scoffing a pork pie and a packet of crisps. Next day, the hangover makes you crave yet more fat and carbs. I do still enjoy a drink but now my first choice is a vodka and slimline tonic instead of a beer – fewer calories. If I overdo it, I try not to drink again for three days and I'm learning to keep control. And my snack of choice these days is Marmite rice cakes!

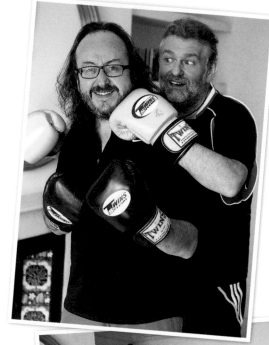

Dave: I never used to count calories. Just wasn't me. Now it's a way of life and I find it helps me be aware of everything I eat. I don't want to waste my calorie budget on a bit of rubbish – better to save myself for something good. I don't stick to the regime all the time but I do eat sensibly and if I find I've put on a pound or two I go back to 1,500 calories a day for a while. When I started this diet, my sugar levels were high and I was in danger of Type 2 diabetes. Now I'm back to a healthy level and I'm determined to stay that way. I've got into the exercise habit and it's something I enjoy and look forward to – I go to the gym and I've got into boxing. I've loads more energy and I find I don't get nearly so tired when we're on the road and filming.

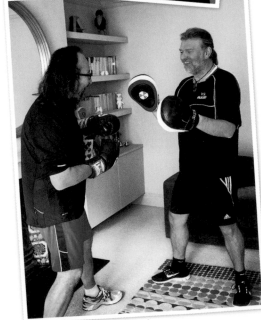

LITTLE THINGS MEAN A LOT

- Break out of old habits – you don't have to have butter on your bread.

- If you fancy a sandwich, make it an open one or a wrap. Lots of topping and less of the stodge equals loads of flavour and fewer calories.

- We drink our coffee black now and we've realised that good coffee doesn't need milk. It spoils the taste.

- Instead of sloshing the oil into the pan we brush it on or use a spray oil. Saves calories and you hardly notice the difference.

- We buy half-fat crème fraiche and half-fat coconut milk. Just as much taste but lower in calories.

- Think about your ingredients. Using low-fat yoghurt in your curry instead of full fat doesn't affect the taste but using fresh spices really does make a difference. Maximise on taste while minimising cals.

- Change the balance of your plate. Make carbs the smallest part of your meal, with lots of vegetables and a modest portion of protein.

- Watch out for the booze. Alcoholic drinks are empty calories and can wipe out your daily calorie allowance in no time. You don't have to go teetotal forever – just while you get your weight under control. Then be careful. Half a pint of lager or bitter is about 100 calories and so is a small (125ml) glass of wine, but most pubs serve larger measures than this so watch out.

BREAKFAST & BRUNCH

"When I'm at home I cook one of the recipes in this book, like poached eggs and smoked salmon or our great light version of kedgeree. I really enjoy these and they're far lower in calories than the breakfasts I used to eat. When I'm on the road it's harder, but my fail-safe option is a calorie-counted cowboy's breakfast – pork and beans! Give me half a can of baked beans on brown toast – no butter – with a couple of slices of ham and I'm happy. Quick, tasty and filling."

Dave

POACHED EGG, SMOKED SALMON AND SPINACH

205 calories per portion

Packed with protein and flavour, this is a prince among breakfasts that will keep you going for hours. Poached eggs have far fewer calories than fried so they make a great guilt-free treat.

Serves 2
Prep: 5 minutes
Cooking time: 5 minutes

1 tsp white wine vinegar
2 very fresh medium eggs
10g butter
100g young spinach leaves. trimmed
   if necessary
good pinch of freshly grated nutmeg
4 slices of smoked salmon
   (about 75g)
flaked sea salt
freshly ground black pepper

Half fill a medium non-stick saucepan with water, add the vinegar and bring it to the boil. Now, don't forget our special tip for perfect poaching. Place the eggs, still in their shells, into the boiling water for precisely 20 seconds. Remove them carefully with a slotted spoon and turn the heat down so the water is simmering gently.

Crack the eggs gently into the water, let them drop to the bottom of the pan and cook for 3 minutes. The water should be gently bubbling and the eggs will rise to the surface when they are nearly ready. If they do stick to the bottom of the pan, give them a gentle nudge with a spoon.

While the eggs are cooking, melt the butter in a large non-stick frying pan over a medium heat. Add the spinach and sprinkle with a grating of nutmeg, salt and freshly ground black pepper.

Cook the spinach for 1–2 minutes, stirring until the leaves are wilted. Divide it between warmed plates and top each pile of spinach with smoked salmon.

Remove the eggs from the simmering water with a slotted spoon, drain briefly and place on top of the smoked salmon. Season with a little extra pepper and serve immediately.

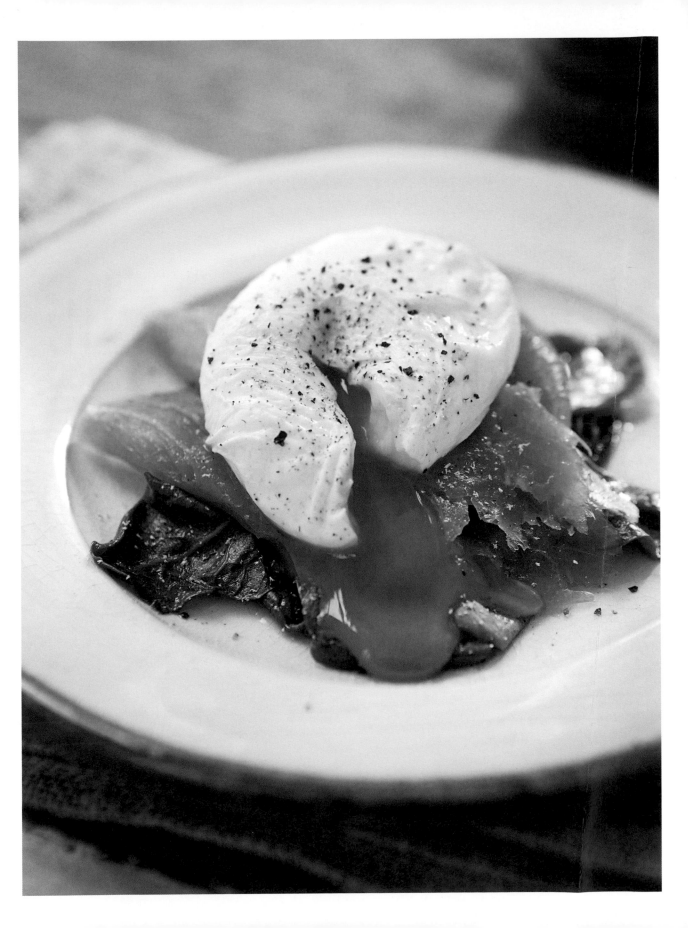

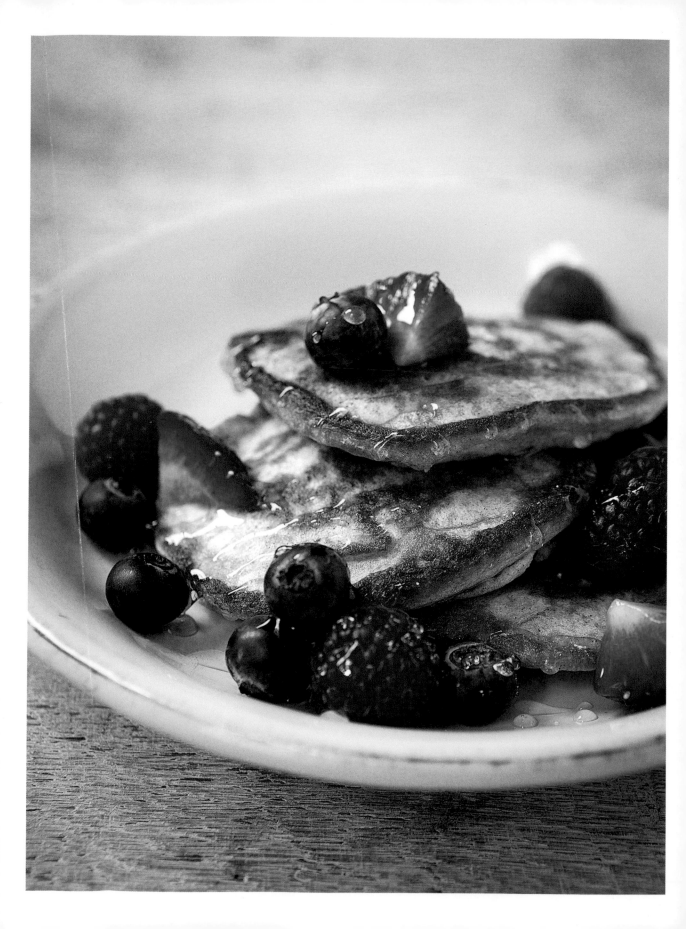

FLUFFY BANANA PANCAKES

251 calories per portion of 3 pancakes with fruit and honey (74 calories per pancake)

The whole family will love these pancakes – and not just for breakfast. They also make a lovely snack served just as they are or warmed through in a toaster. It's tempting to slather them with butter, but resist or your calorie count will go through the roof!

Sift the flour, baking powder and cinnamon, if using, into a large bowl. Whisk the egg whites in a separate bowl until stiff but not dry and whisk in the caster sugar.

Stir the milk slowly and gradually into the flour mixture, then beat hard with a metal whisk to get rid of any lumps. Peel the banana, cut it in half lengthways, then into thin slices. Stir the banana slices into the pancake batter.

Fold a quarter of the whisked egg whites into the pancake batter with a large metal spoon until evenly combined, then very gently fold in the rest. You want to try to keep as much air in the pancakes as possible, so they are light and fluffy when you cook them.

Brush a large non-stick frying pan with a little oil and place it over a medium-high heat. Add 4 large spoonfuls of the pancake batter to the pan, spacing them well apart.

Cook the pancakes for 1½ –2 minutes on one side, until the surface looks almost dry and you can see small air bubbles rising to the surface. Flip the pancakes over and cook on the other side for another 2 minutes until they're puffed up and lightly browned.

Pop the pancakes on to a plate and keep them warm while you cook the rest in the same way. Serve the hot pancakes with lots of fresh berries and just a dribble of agave syrup, honey or golden syrup.

Makes 12
Prep: 10 minutes
Cooking time: 12 minutes

175g self-raising flour
½ tsp baking powder
½ tsp ground cinnamon (optional)
2 large egg whites
1 tbsp caster sugar
225ml semi-skimmed milk
1 ripe, medium banana
1 tsp sunflower oil, for frying
200g mixed fresh berries, such
    as raspberries, blueberries,
    redcurrants and strawberries
4 tsp agave nectar, honey or
    golden syrup

AWESOME OATS

Oats are a slow-release carb so they keep you going for longer and make a cracking breakfast with some poached fruit, low-fat yoghurt and other delicious things. Here are a few of our favourite ways of getting our oats.

Serves 2
Prep: 5 minutes
Cooking time: 3–5 minutes

60g porridge oats
¼ tsp ground cinnamon (optional)
350ml semi-skimmed milk
100ml water
1 small banana
10g pecan nuts (6 or 7 halves)
1 tbsp maple syrup

BANANA AND PECAN PORRIDGE

285 calories per portion

Put the porridge oats in a medium non-stick saucepan with the cinnamon, if using, milk and water and place over a medium heat. Cook for 3–5 minutes or until the oats are tender and creamy, stirring frequently. Pour the porridge into 2 bowls. Add some slices of banana, scatter with a few pecan nuts, breaking them up roughly, and drizzle with maple syrup.

Serves 2–3
Prep: 5 minutes, plus soaking

50g porridge oats
25g blanched hazelnuts, chopped
1 eating apple
75ml apple juice
100ml semi-skimmed milk
150g fat-free yoghurt
1 tbsp light brown sugar
   or runny honey
200g fresh mixed berries, to serve

BIRCHER MUESLI

328 calories per portion (if serving 2); 219 calories per portion (if serving 3)

Put the oats and hazelnuts in a bowl. Peel the apple and grate it coarsely, then stir the grated apple and apple juice into the oats. Stir in the milk, yoghurt and sugar or honey until well mixed. Cover and chill for 1 hour or overnight. Serve the muesli topped with mixed berries and enjoy.

Serves 2
Prep: 5 minutes

75g jumbo porridge oats
25g luxury mixed dried fruit
15g flaked almonds
50g fresh blueberries
150ml semi-skimmed milk
3 tbsp low-fat natural yoghurt
1 tbsp runny honey (optional)

HOME-MADE MUESLI

303 calories per portion

Divide the oats, dried fruit and flaked almonds between 2 bowls – toast the almonds if you have time. Scatter the blueberries on top and serve with milk and low-fat yoghurt. Add a drizzle of honey if using.

PORRIDGE WITH SPICED PLUMS

258 calories per portion

Serves 2
Prep: 5 minutes
Cooking time: 8–10 minutes

Put the plums and sugar in a microwavable bowl. Break the star anise in half and drop it on top. Sprinkle with the cinnamon and toss everything together lightly. Cover the top of the bowl and microwave on high for about 2 minutes. Stir the plums, cover and microwave on high for another 1–2 minutes or until the plums are softened and juicy but still holding their shape. If you prefer, put the plums, sugar and spices in a saucepan with 4 tablespoons of water. Bring to a gentle simmer and cook for 5 minutes, stirring gently

Put the porridge oats in a medium non-stick saucepan with the milk and water and place over a medium heat. Cook for 3–5 minutes or until the oats are tender and creamy, stirring frequently. Pour the porridge into 2 bowls and top with the spiced plums and any juice. Add a spoonful of yoghurt and a pinch of grated nutmeg to each bowl if you like. (Watch that you don't eat the star anise!)

2 large red or black plums, quartered
   and stones removed
1 tbsp caster or light brown sugar
1 star anise
good pinch of ground cinnamon
60g porridge oats
350ml semi-skimmed milk
100ml water
2 large tbsp low-fat yoghurt
finely grated nutmeg (optional)

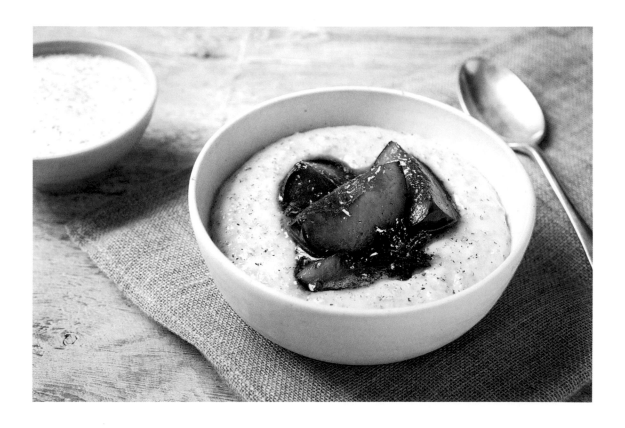

SCRAMBLED EGG WITH BACON AND MUSHROOMS

337 calories per portion

Almost like a full English, this version has far fewer calories. It's still delicious though and great for a Sunday brunch. You could serve some slices of boiled ham instead of bacon if you like, and save even more calories.

Serves 2
Prep: 5 minutes
Cooking time: 5 minutes

1 tsp sunflower oil
125g small chestnut mushrooms, wiped and halved (or sliced if large)
2 rashers of rindless lean smoked back bacon
15g butter
4 large eggs
flaked sea salt
freshly ground black pepper

Heat the oil in a large non-stick frying pan over a high heat. Add the mushrooms and stir fry for 1 minute until lightly browned.

Push the mushrooms to one side of the pan and add the bacon to the other. Reduce the heat and cook the bacon for 2 minutes on each side until lightly browned.

While the mushrooms and bacon are cooking, melt the butter in a medium non-stick saucepan. Beat the eggs with a metal whisk until smooth and season with salt and pepper.

Tip the eggs into the saucepan and cook them over a low heat for 2 minutes, stirring regularly until lightly set.

Divide the scrambled egg between the warmed plates, add the mushrooms and top with the bacon. Serve immediately.

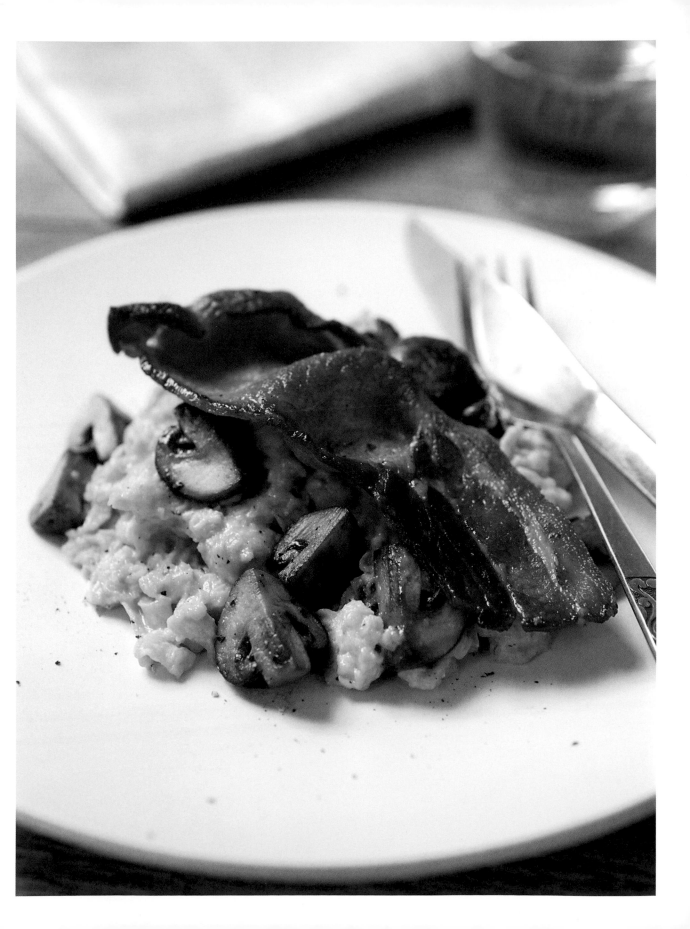

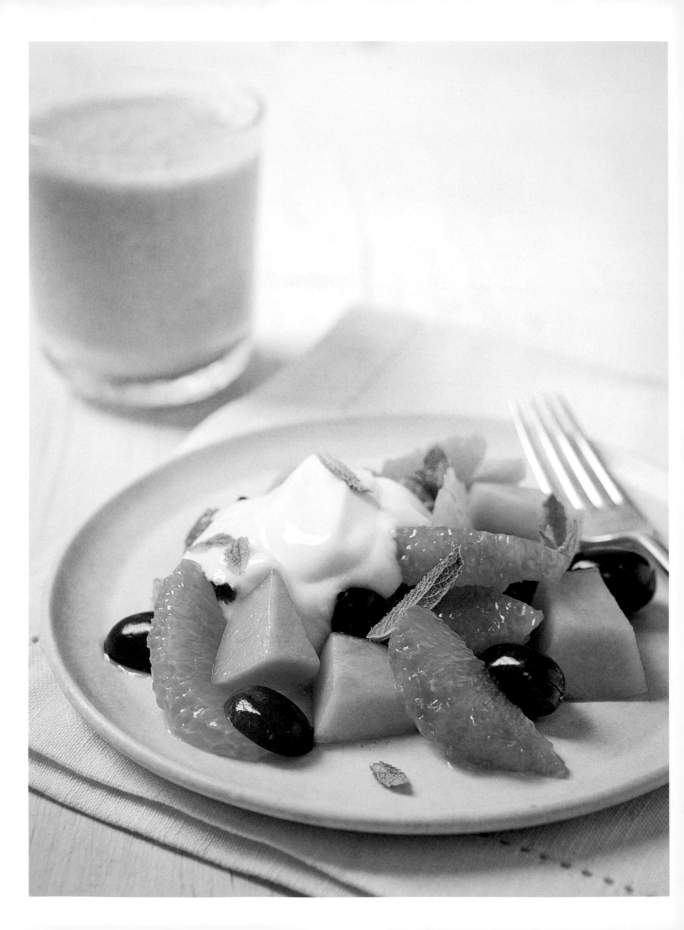

WAKEY WAKEY BREAKFAST SALAD

95 calories per portion

Packed with sparky fresh citrus, this salad really does put some zip in your pip. It keeps well in the fridge, so make it the night before if you like and get a head start on your day

Slice the ends off the grapefruit and place it on a chopping board, resting it on one of the cut sides. Using a small sharp knife, cut off the peel and pith, working your way around the fruit. Next, cut between the membranes to release the segments. Put the segments in a salad bowl along with any juice on your board. Do the same thing with 2 of the oranges.

Cut the melon half into 6 wedges and scoop out the seeds. Slide a knife between the flesh and the skin, chuck out the skin and cut the melon flesh into 2.5cm pieces. Or if you want to be really fancy, use a melon baller to scoop out the fruit. Add the melon to the citrus fruits and scatter over the grapes and mint leaves.

Cut the remaining orange in half, squeeze out the juice and pour it over the salad. Toss lightly and serve with low-fat natural yoghurt.

Serves 4
Prep: 15 minutes

———————————

1 ruby or pink grapefruit

3 large oranges

½ cantaloupe melon (about 450g unskinned)

200g red seedless grapes, rinsed and halved if large

20 small fresh mint leaves

150ml low-fat natural yoghurt, for serving

GOOD MORNING SMOOTHIE

143 calories per 250ml portion

Hull and wash the strawberries and peel and slice the bananas. Put the strawberries in a food processor or blender with the bananas, milk, yoghurt and oats.

Blitz until as smooth as possible, then divide the mixture between 4 glasses and serve.

Serves 4
Makes: 1 litre
Prep: 5 minutes

———————————

300g fresh strawberries

2 large ripe bananas

300ml semi-skimmed milk, well chilled

150g fat-free natural yoghurt

2 tbsp porridge oats

LIGHT KEDGEREE

436 calories per portion (if serving 4); 290 calories per portion (if serving 6)

Our light yet creamy-tasting version of this classic is guaranteed to satisfy the most discerning of dieters. And kedgeree is not just for breakfast. It makes a great supper dish too.

Serves 4–6
Prep: 20 minutes
Cooking time: 25–30 minutes

300ml semi-skimmed milk
500ml water
pinch of saffron strands
350g smoked haddock fillets
   (unskinned and preferably
   undyed), cut in half
oil, for spraying
1 medium onion, finely chopped
4 medium eggs, fridge cold
2 tsp hot curry powder
250g easy-cook long-grain rice
   (such as Uncle Ben's)
75g frozen peas
15g bunch of flatleaf or curly parsley
freshly ground black pepper

Pour the milk and water into a large non-stick saucepan and stir in the saffron. Add the fish, skin-side up, then bring to a simmer and immediately turn off the heat. Cover the pan with a lid and leave the fish to poach for 5 minutes. Bring a kettle of water to the boil.

Meanwhile, mist the base of a large non-stick saucepan with oil and place it over a medium heat. Add the onion, cover with a lid and fry gently for 5 minutes until softened and golden, stirring occasionally. Remove the fish with a slotted spatula and put it on a plate, skin-side up. Pour the poaching milk into a wide jug.

Half fill a medium pan with just-boiled water from the kettle and bring it back to the boil. Gently add the eggs, bring the water to the boil and cook for 9 minutes.

Stir the curry powder into the pan with the onion and cook for 30 seconds, stirring. Add the rice and cook for a few seconds, then pour in the poaching milk and bring it to a gentle simmer. Cook for 10 minutes, stirring regularly, especially towards the end of the cooking time.

Add the peas to the pan with the rice and continue cooking and stirring regularly over a low heat for another 3–4 minutes until the rice is tender and almost all the liquid is absorbed. If the rice isn't quite cooked after this time, add a little extra water and continue cooking for 2–3 minutes more. Drain the eggs under cold running water until they are cool enough to handle.

Strip the skin off the haddock and flake the flesh into large chunks, getting rid of any bones that you may come across. Save a few of the parsley sprigs for garnishing the kedgeree and roughly chop the rest.

Stir the cooked haddock, parsley and lots of black pepper into the rice and peas, taking care not to break up the fish too much. Warm through over a low heat for 1–2 minutes until the fish is hot. Peel the eggs, cut them into quarters and dot over the rice. Scatter a few parsley leaves on top and serve right away.

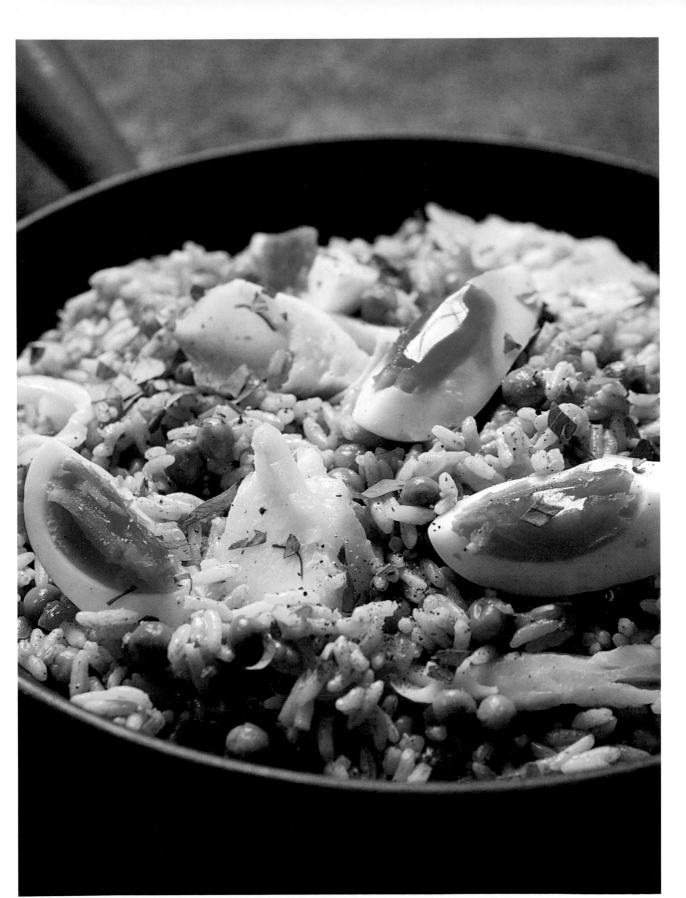

BANANA AND SULTANA MUFFINS

119 calories per muffin

Muffins on a diet – surely not! But yes, you can feel free to stuff in a muffin. These little beauties are lower in fat and sugar than the standard and still nicely naughty. They don't have the same texture as a shop-bought muffin, but they are tasty and filling.

Makes 12
Prep: 15 minutes
Cooking time: 20 minutes

oil, for spraying (optional)
250g self-raising flour
1 tsp ground cinnamon
1 tsp bicarbonate of soda
finely grated zest of 1 lemon
2 very ripe medium bananas, about 100g peeled weight each
250ml semi-skimmed milk
75g sultanas
3 medium egg whites
1 tbsp golden caster sugar

Preheat the oven to 210°C/Fan 190°C/Gas 6½. Line a 12-hole, deep muffin tin with non-stick paper cases or folded squares of baking parchment. If you don't have any paper cases or baking parchment, spray the holes of your muffin tin with oil.

Sift the flour, cinnamon and bicarbonate of soda into a large bowl and stir in the lemon zest. Make a well in the centre. Mash the bananas with a fork until they're almost smooth and stir in the milk. Pour this mixture on to the flour and mix with a large metal whisk until lightly combined. Stir in the sultanas.

In a separate bowl, whisk the egg whites with an electric whisk until stiff peaks form. Fold the beaten egg whites quickly and lightly into the batter using a large metal spoon.

Working quickly, divide the batter between the muffin cases. Sprinkle with the golden caster sugar to give the muffins a nice crunchy topping.

Bake the muffins for 20 minutes, until they're well risen and golden brown. Serve warm or leave them to cool on a wire rack if you can bear to wait that long! Store in an airtight container and eat within 2 days. You can reheat the muffins for a few seconds in a microwave if you like, but don't overdo it or they'll be tough.

Because these muffins are very low in fat you might find they stick to the paper cases a bit, but don't worry, you won't lose too much.

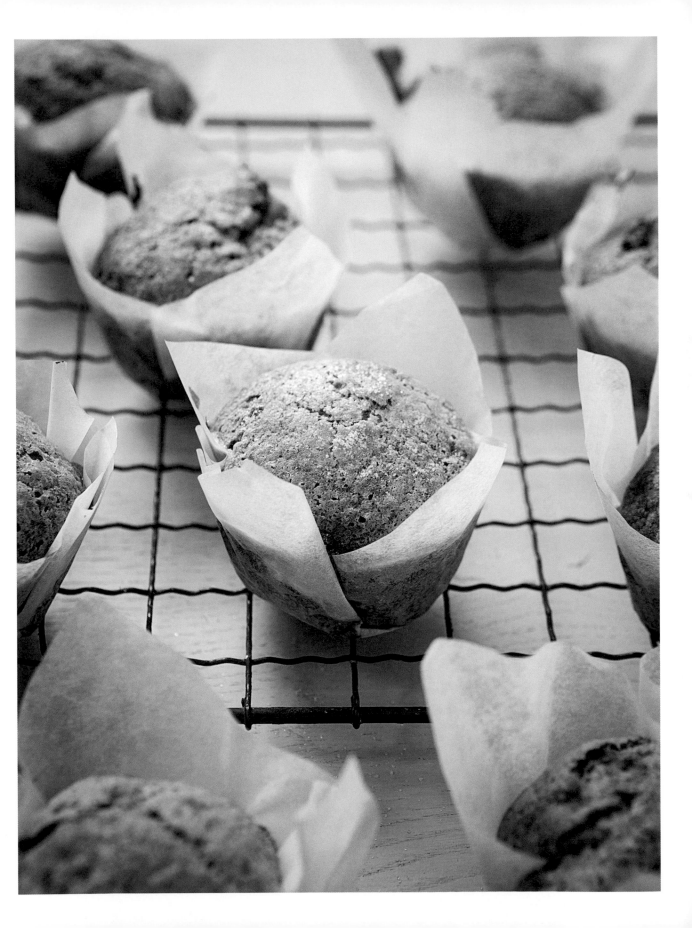

REAL FOOD FAST

"You know the feeling. You get in after a long day and you're starving. You want something quick and you reach for the pasta or a ready meal or start scoffing hunks of bread and butter. Next thing you know your calorie budget is broken. Don't despair – you can put together a fast, nourishing meal for the family in less time than you think. Cook up our five-minute pizza, chicken fajitas or griddled lamb steaks and you'll have resisted the temptation to snack, slaked your hunger and stuck to the diet. Everyone's a winner."

Si

FIVE-MINUTE PIZZA

250 calories per pizza

Our super-quick pizza is based on a tortilla wrap instead of pizza dough, which makes it lower in calories and fast to prepare – a pizz-a genius! We like to add some pitted olives to our pizza before grilling but don't forget that every 15 grams of olives ups the calorie count by 15.

Makes 1 pizza (serves 1)
Prep: 3½ minutes
Cooking time: 1½ minutes

1 large flour tortilla wrap
3 tbsp passata with basil
20g wafer-thin ham
   (a couple of slices)
2 good pinches of dried oregano
20g half-fat Cheddar cheese, finely
   grated
small handful of rocket or
   baby salad leaves
½ tsp extra virgin olive oil
½ tsp good balsamic vinegar
   (optional)
olives in brine (optional)
freshly ground black pepper

Preheat the grill to its hottest setting. Place the tortilla on a baking sheet and spread with the passata, leaving a 2cm gap around the edge.

Tear the ham into strips and arrange them on top of the tortilla. Sprinkle with the oregano and then the grated Cheddar. Season with black pepper.

Toss the rocket or salad leaves with olive oil and a dribble of balsamic vinegar if you like. Put to one side.

Place the pizza under the grill and cook for about 1½ minutes or until the cheese has melted and the edges of the pizza are beginning to brown. Watch carefully so it doesn't burn! Slide the pizza on to a board or a warmed plate, top with the salad and serve immediately.

By the way, passata is sieved Italian tomatoes and we reckon it's really useful stuff. You'll find it in cans, jars or cartons in the supermarket. Use any leftover passata in a sauce, such as Bolognese.

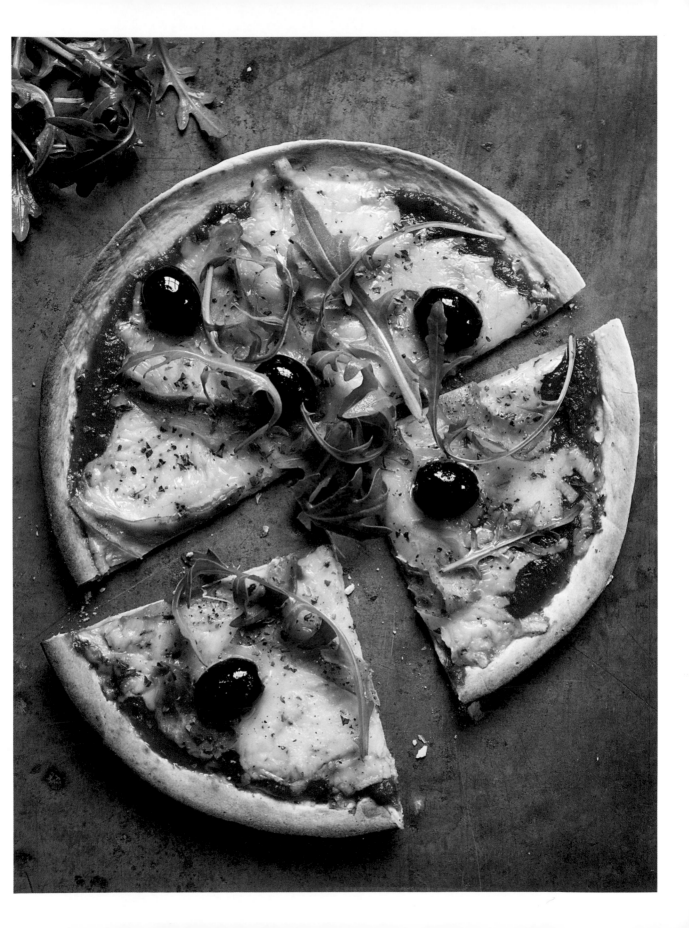

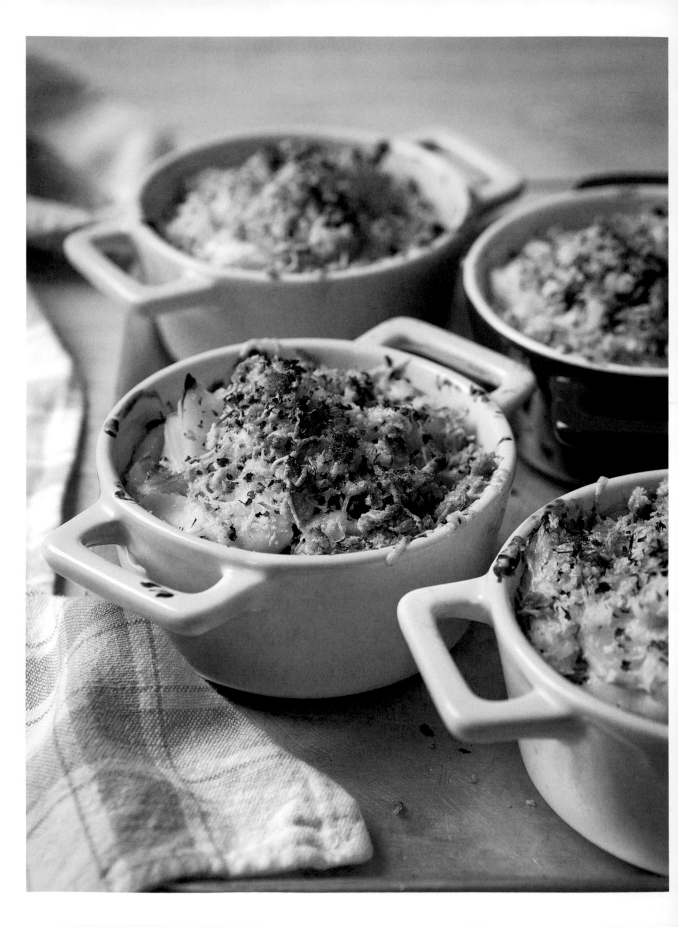

CREAMY HADDOCK WITH BROCCOLI

281 calories per portion

These little pots of loveliness are deliciously creamy and comforting – just right for a winter supper. Using smoked haddock as well as fresh adds extra flavour and the broccoli bulks the dish out while keeping the calorie count low.

Place 4 small, shallow flameproof dishes on a baking tray. To make the gratin topping, mix the breadcrumbs, cheese and parsley in a bowl, then set aside while you prepare the filling.

Mix 4 tablespoons of the milk with the cornflour in a small bowl until smooth and set aside. Pour the rest of the milk into a large non-stick saucepan and add the onion, bay leaf and lemon peel. Cut the fish fillets in half, place them skin-side down in the pan and bring to a gentle simmer over a medium heat. Cook for 3 minutes, basting the fish occasionally with the milk until only just cooked. Cover the pan with a lid and leave to stand for 5 minutes. During the standing time the fish will continue to cook, so it's important not to simmer it for too long first. Preheat the oven to 220°C/Fan 200°C/Gas 7.

While the fish is cooking, half fill a small pan with water and bring it to the boil. Add the broccoli florets, bring the water back to the boil and cook for 2 minutes. Drain the broccoli, then rinse in a sieve under cold running water until cool and drain again.

Place a colander over a clean non-stick saucepan and drain the fish, collecting the milk in the pan. Stir the cornflour mixture into the warm milk and heat gently over a medium heat until it has thickened, stirring constantly. Bring the sauce to a simmer and continue stirring until it's smooth and thick. Stir in the cheese and mustard, then cook over a low heat for another 2–3 minutes, stirring. Season with salt and freshly ground black pepper to taste and stir in the broccoli florets.

Flake the fish into chunky pieces and chuck away the skin, onion, bay leaf and lemon peel. Add the fish to the pan with the sauce and stir once or twice. Try not to break up the fish too much.

Divide the fish mixture between the dishes. Sprinkle with the gratin mixture and bake for 15–20 minutes or until the tops are nicely browned, the fish is hot and the sauce is bubbling.

Serves 4
Prep: 15 minutes
Cooking time: 25–30 minutes

600ml semi-skimmed milk
5 tbsp cornflour
1 small onion, cut into 6 wedges
1 bay leaf
2 long strips of lemon peel
200g smoked haddock fillet (unskinned and preferably undyed)
250g thick fresh haddock or cod fillet (unskinned)
300g broccoli, trimmed and cut into small florets
20g Gruyère cheese, finely grated
1 tsp prepared English mustard
flaked sea salt
freshly ground black pepper

Gratin topping
15g fresh white breadcrumbs
10g Gruyère cheese, finely grated
½ tsp dried parsley

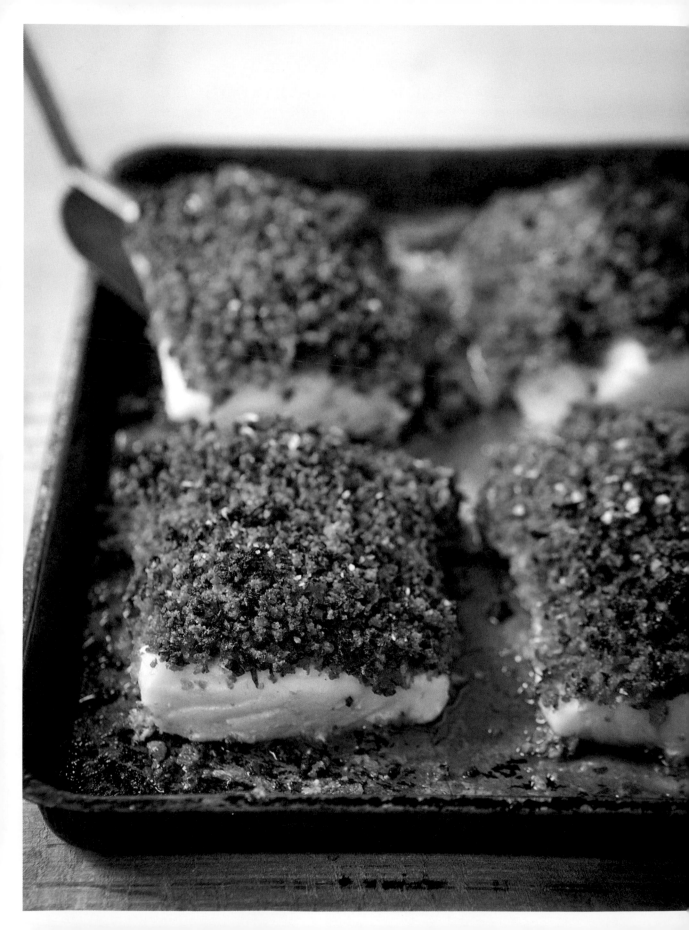

BAKED FISH WITH CHORIZO CRUST

255 calories per portion

There's no doubt about it – chorizo is full of fat and calories. But we love it and it has such a great flavour that a little goes a long way. This is a version of a recipe we first cooked on a beach in Patagonia, but with a lower calorie count. Different types of chorizo vary in calories, but the lower-calorie versions will be about 300 calories per 100g, so choose those if you can.

Put the fish in a non-metallic bowl and sprinkle the lime juice over it. Toss lightly, then cover and chill while you make the crust.

Lightly mist a medium non-stick frying pan with oil and fry the chorizo over a medium heat for 1–2 minutes or until the fat begins to run, stirring regularly. Tear the bread into pieces (you should have about 65g after you've removed the crusts) and add it to the pan. Toss the bread with the chorizo and cook for 3 minutes more until the pieces are stained all over with the red fat, stirring. Tip it all on to a plate and leave to cool for 10 minutes. Preheat the oven to 200°C/Fan 180°C/Gas 6.

Transfer the bread and chorizo to a food processor and blitz into crumbs. Add the garlic, lime zest, parsley, Parmesan, a teaspoon of the salt and lots of freshly ground black pepper, then process again to combine the ingredients thoroughly.

Lightly mist a baking tray with oil and put the fish, skin-side down, on the tray with the marinating juices. Spoon the chorizo mixture on top of the fish fillets and press it on firmly. Bake for 15–18 minutes until the fish is cooked and the crust is crisp.

Put the fish on warm plates, drizzle with the olive oil and sprinkle with a little more salt if you like. Serve with lime wedges for squeezing. This fish goes very well with our creamy mash (see page 180) and a few green beans, sugar snap peas or other green vegetables.

Serves 4
Prep: 10 minutes
Cooking time: 20 minutes

---

4 x 150g thick white fish fillets, such as haddock or cod, skinned
freshly squeezed juice and finely grated zest of ½ large lime
oil, for spraying
100g chorizo sausage, skinned (if necessary) and cut into 1.5cm slices
2 thick slices day-old white bread (about 100g), crusts removed
1 garlic clove, finely sliced
15g bunch of flatleaf parsley, leaves roughly chopped
1 tbsp finely grated Parmesan cheese
1 tsp flaked sea salt, plus extra for seasoning
2 tsp extra virgin olive oil
extra lime wedges, to serve
freshly ground black pepper

TURKEY BURGERS AND CHIPS

313 calories per portion

These have that lovely, juicy mouth-feel of a trad burger, but as they're made with turkey they're much lower in calories than the usual beef. You can make them with chicken as well. The chips look and taste the business but are made with a tiny amount of oil.

Serves 4
Prep: 20 minutes
Cooking time: 25 minutes

4 tsp sunflower oil
2 slender leeks, each about 125g, trimmed and finely sliced
1 medium courgette (about 150g), trimmed and finely grated
500g minced turkey breast
finely grated zest of ½ lemon
½ tsp flaked sea salt
6 tbsp tomato relish, to serve
large mixed salad, to serve
freshly ground black pepper

Paprika chips
3 medium potatoes (about 475g)
1 tsp sunflower oil
½ tsp paprika
½ tsp flaked sea salt
freshly ground black pepper

Preheat the oven to 220°C/Fan 200°C/Gas 7 and get all the ingredients ready for your burgers.

To prepare the chips, peel the potatoes and cut each one into 8–10 long wedges. Put the wedges in a bowl and toss with the oil, then sprinkle with paprika, salt and black pepper. Scatter the chips over a baking tray and cook for 20–25 minutes until tender and lightly browned, turning them halfway through the cooking time.

While the potatoes are cooking, make the burgers. Heat 2 teaspoons of the oil in a large non-stick frying pan and fry the leeks very gently for 3 minutes until softened but not coloured, stirring regularly. Tip the leeks into a large bowl and leave to cool for 5 minutes. Add the grated courgette, minced turkey, lemon zest, salt and lots of black pepper to the leeks, then get in there and mix it all well with your hands until thoroughly combined. Form the mince mixture into 8 balls and flatten them into burger shapes.

Brush the remaining oil over a baking tray, place the burgers on the tray and bake them on the shelf above the potatoes for 5 minutes. Carefully turn them over with tongs and cook for a further 5 minutes or until lightly browned and thoroughly cooked. If you prefer, you could cook the burgers in a frying pan, lightly misted with oil. Fry them for about 5 minutes on each side or until thoroughly cooked.

Serve the burgers hot with the chips, salad and relish.

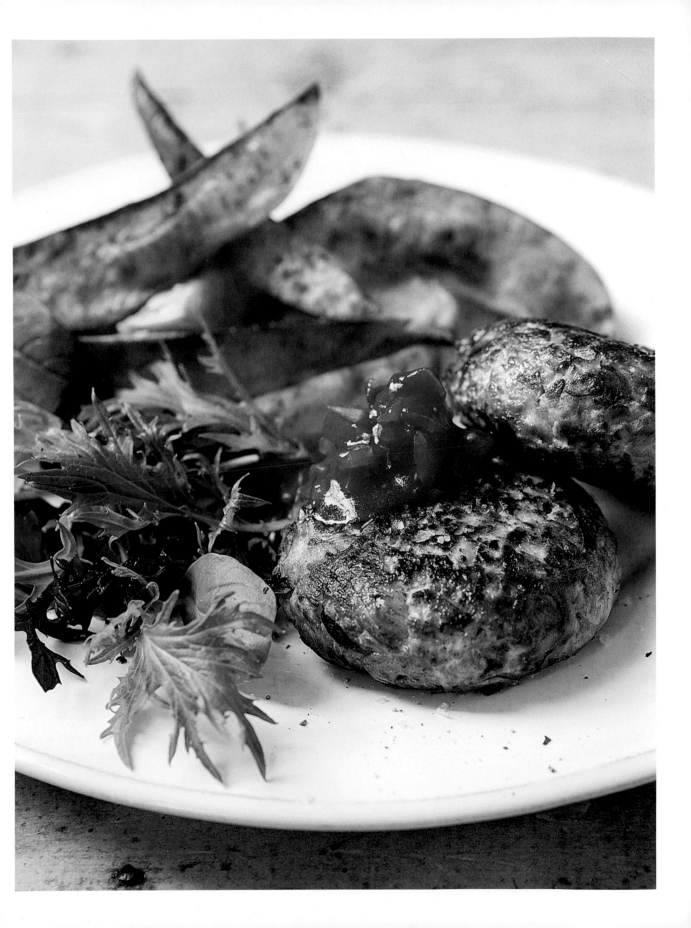

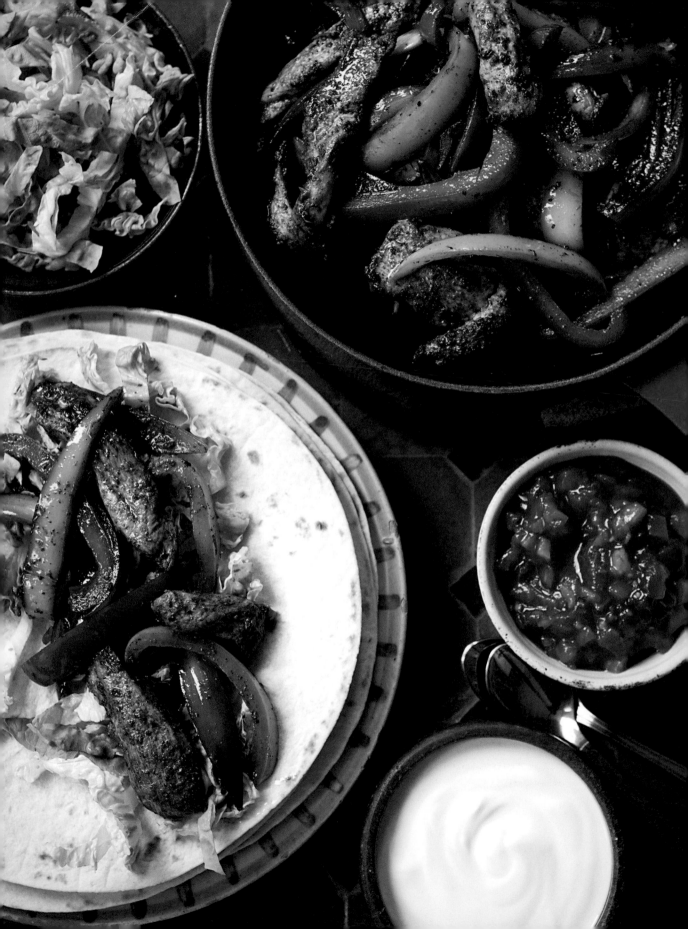

FAST CHICKEN FAJITAS

443 calories per portion

Spicy salsa, chilli and lime give these a real Mexican wave of flavour and everyone will enjoy getting round the table and putting their fajitas together. A lovely dish to share with family and friends.

Trim off any visible fat from the chicken breasts, then cut them into thin strips and put these in a bowl. Pour over the lime juice and sprinkle with the cumin, coriander, oregano and chilli powder. Season with salt and black pepper and toss well.

Put the shredded lettuce, crème fraiche and salsa in separate bowls.

Heat the oil in a large non-stick frying pan over a medium-high heat. Stir-fry the marinated chicken for 3 minutes over a medium-high heat until lightly browned, stirring to scrape any spices off the bottom of the pan. Tip the chicken on to a plate.

Put the pan back on the heat and add the peppers and onion. Stir-fry for a few seconds then add the 3 tablespoons of cold water and steam-fry for 3 minutes more until the veg are beginning to soften and lightly brown.

Put the chicken back in the pan and cook with the vegetables for 1–2 minutes more until cooked through – check that no pinkness remains. While the chicken and vegetables are frying, heat the tortillas according to the packet instructions.

Serve the warm tortillas topped with shredded lettuce, sizzling chicken and vegetables from the pan, tomato salsa and half-fat crème fraiche. Season with an extra squeeze of lime if you like.

By the way, we think that steam-frying, as above, is a great way to cook food without too much fat. First fry the food in an open pan with only a little oil – just enough to add some colour to vegetables or seal meat, then add a few tablespoons of liquid such as water or stock. The hot liquid will create steam and continue to cook the food without the need for extra fat to prevent it sticking. Try it next time you are making a stir-fry or softening some vegetables for a casserole.

Serves 4
Prep: 20 minutes
Cooking time: 8–10 minutes

3 boneless, skinless chicken breasts
   (each about 150g)
freshly squeezed juice of ½ lime
1½ tsp ground cumin
1½ tsp ground coriander
1 tsp dried oregano
½ tsp hot chilli powder
2 little gem lettuces, trimmed and
   finely shredded
3 tbsp half-fat crème fraiche
8 tbsp ready-made fresh tomato
   salsa dip
1 tbsp sunflower oil
1 yellow pepper, deseeded and sliced
1 red pepper, deseeded and sliced
1 medium red onion, cut into
   12 wedges
3 tbsp cold water
8 small flour tortillas
lime wedges, for squeezing
   (optional)
flaked sea salt
freshly ground black pepper

QUICK CHICKEN CORDON BLEU

293 calories per portion

Look at this – do you reckon it looks like diet food? We don't. This recipe is the ultimate speedy family supper. We've called it Cordon Bleu, as it contains the traditional melted Swiss cheese and ham, but our version isn't coated with breadcrumbs or deep-fried, so it's lower in fat and calories. And to make it super easy we use ready-sliced Emmental and good-quality ham from a packet.

Serves 4
Prep: 10 minutes
Cooking time: 10–14 minutes

4 boneless, skinless chicken breasts
   (each about 150g)
4 thin slices of ham (each about
   35g, not the wafer-thin stuff)
4 thin slices of Emmental cheese
   (each about 25g)
oil, for spraying
flaked sea salt
freshly ground black pepper

Put a chicken breast on a board and turn it over so the smooth side is underneath. Using a sharp knife, carefully cut horizontally through the breast from the curved side almost all the way through to the other side and open it out like a book. You may need to go a little way, then gently flip the chicken open and carry on gently cutting through the meat with a knife so it opens easily without tearing. It should have a heart shape when you have finished.

Place the chicken breast between 2 sheets of cling film and flatten it by bashing with a rolling pin until it's about 5mm thick all over. Take care as you bash so the chicken doesn't get too thin and go into holes. Remove the cling film from the top.

Place a slice of ham over the open chicken breast, cut a slice of the cheese in half and place both pieces on one side of the breast. Fold the other side of the ham and the chicken back over to completely enclose the filling. Season the chicken on both sides generously with salt and pepper and set aside. Prepare the other chicken breasts in the same way.

Preheat the oven to 200°C/Fan 180°C/Gas 6. Mist a large non-stick frying pan with oil and place it over a medium heat. When the pan is hot, take the chicken breasts off the cling film, add them to the pan and fry for 3–4 minutes on each side until golden. You may need to fry the chicken in a couple of batches if your pan isn't large enough for all 4 breasts. Transfer the breasts to a baking tray and bake them in the oven for 5–6 minutes until thoroughly cooked.

There should be no pinkness remaining in the chicken meat when you cut it. If you do notice any, pop the chicken back into the oven for a couple of minutes more. Serve the chicken with a large mixed salad and a few new potatoes.

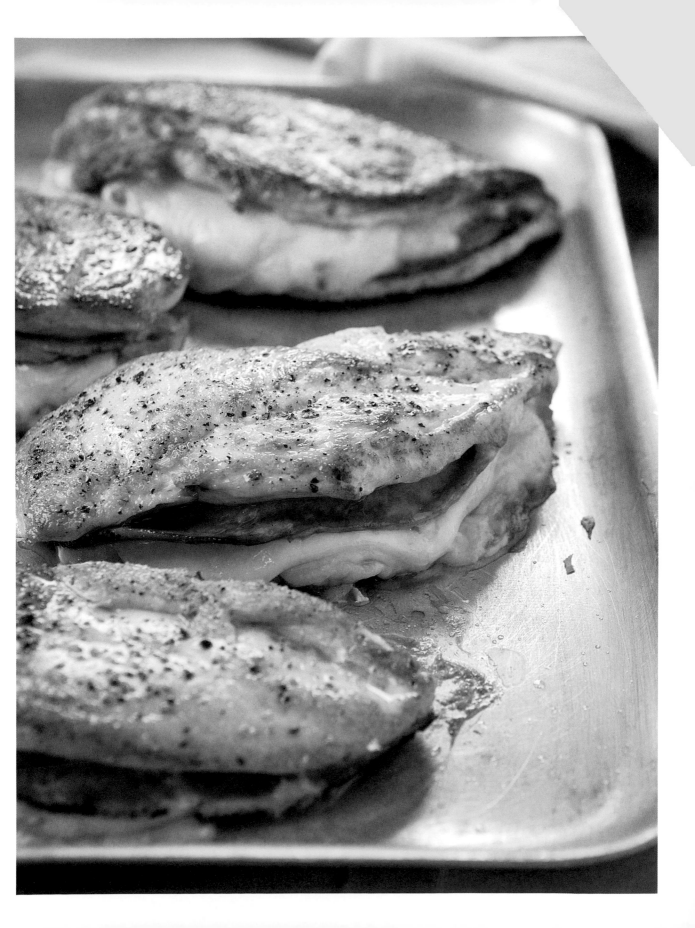

SAUSAGES AND RICH ONION GRAVY

242 calories per portion

Thank goodness, we can still have a dash of the bangers and mash our mothers used to make. If you choose lean sausages and cook with the minimum of fat, there's no reason why you shouldn't include this tasty dish on your menu and still drop the pounds. Look for sausages containing about 100 calories each and make sure they're good quality for the best taste.

Serves 4
Prep: 10 minutes
Cooking time: 20 minutes

½ tsp sunflower oil
8 lean pork sausages
1½ medium onions, thinly sliced
300ml beef stock, made with ½ beef
  stock cube
2 tbsp tomato ketchup
1 tbsp Worcestershire sauce
2 tsp cornflour
1 tbsp cold water
flaked sea salt
freshly ground black pepper

Brush a large non-stick frying pan or sauté pan with the sunflower oil and fry the sausages over a medium heat for 5 minutes, turning occasionally until they're golden brown all over. Add the onions to the pan, turn down the heat slightly and fry for 8–10 minutes or until the sausages are cooked and the onions are softened and golden brown, stirring regularly.

Pour the stock into the pan, add the ketchup and Worcestershire sauce and bring to a simmer. Cook for 3 minutes, stirring occasionally.

Mix the cornflour with the cold water in a small bowl until smooth. Stir this mixture into the pan with the sausages and return to a simmer, then cook for 1–2 minutes more until the sauce is thickened, stirring. Season to taste with salt and pepper and serve with our lower-cal colcannon (see page 181).

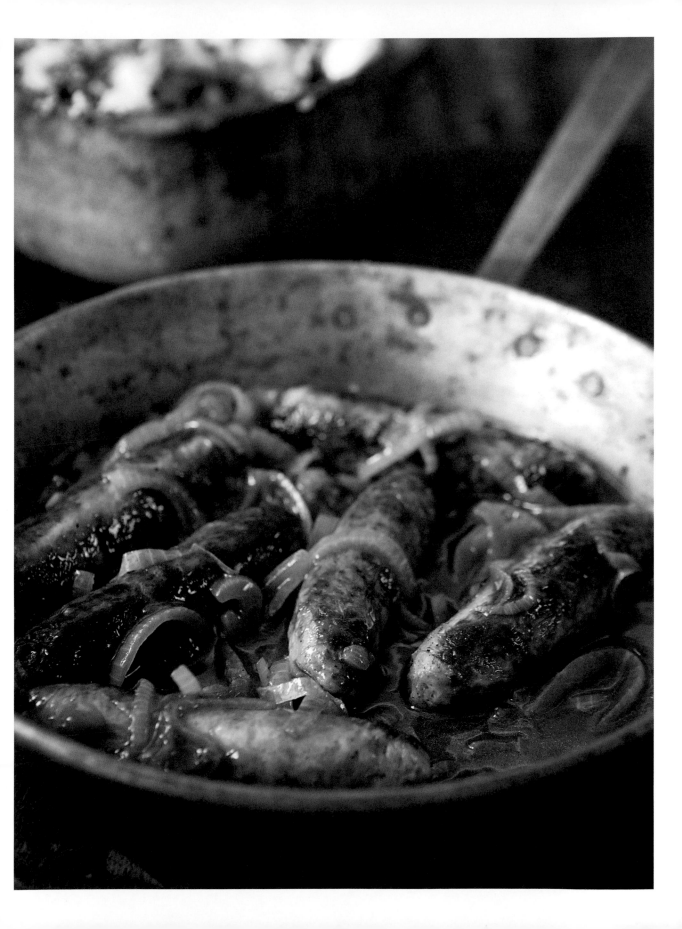

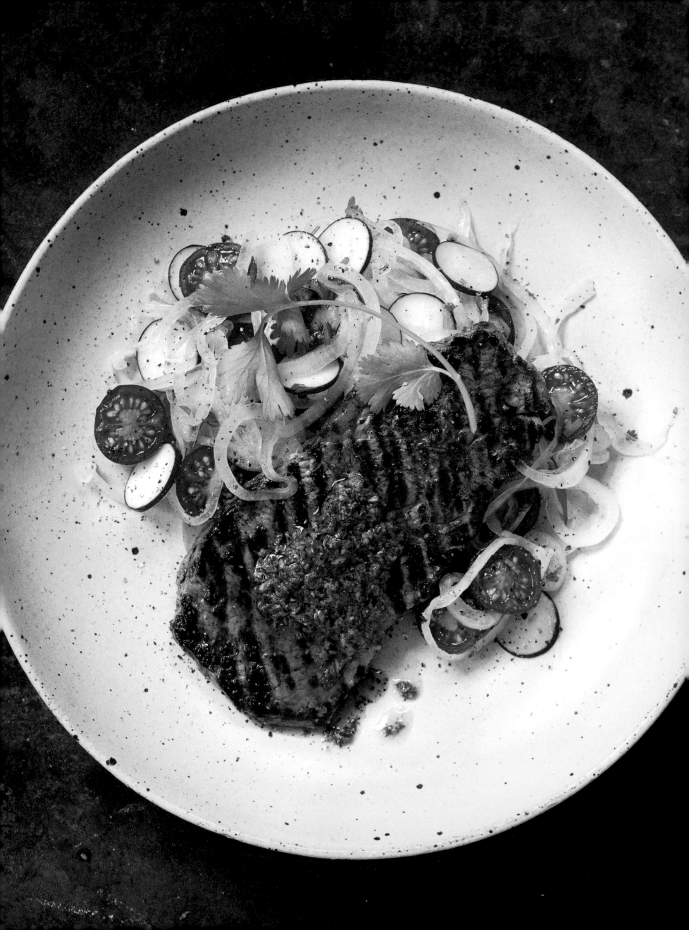

ARGENTINIAN-STYLE STEAK WITH ONION AND RADISH SALAD

249 calories per portion

Even gauchos need to lose a few pounds sometimes. Tangy chimichurri sauce makes this a really special dish and it's served with a great salad. The secret of the salad is to blanch the onion rings before adding them to the salad to take away any bitterness.

To make the chimichurri sauce, strip the leaves from the parsley and put them in a food processor. Add the chopped chilli, garlic, dried oregano, wine vinegar, water and olive oil. Blitz until as finely blended as possible – you may need to remove the lid and push the mixture down a couple of times with a rubber spatula. (If you don't have a food processor, chop the parsley, chilli and garlic very finely and mix with the oregano, vinegar, water and oil.)

Spoon the sauce into a bowl, cover and leave to stand for at least 30 minutes (and up to 3 or 4 hours if you have the time) to allow the flavours to mingle and develop.

For the salad, peel the onions and cut them into rings. Place these in a bowl and pour over enough just-boiled water to cover, then leave to stand for 15 minutes. This takes away any bitterness and heat.

Drain the onion rings and plunge them into cold water. Shake them dry and put them in a bowl with the radishes and tomatoes. Roughly chop the coriander leaves and toss them with the vegetables. Season with salt and lots of black pepper.

Trim off as much fat as possible from the beef. Mist the steaks on both sides with oil and season well with salt and pepper. Heat a non-stick griddle or large frying pan over a very high heat – these steaks are also great cooked on the barbecue.

Cook the steaks for just 30–40 seconds on each side until nicely browned on the outside but still nice and juicy in the middle. You may need to do this in a couple of batches. Serve hot with the onion and radish salad and chimichurri sauce for spooning over.

Serves 4
Prep: 20 minutes, plus standing time
Cooking time: about 1 minute

4 x 100g lean, thin-cut frying steaks
oil, for spraying
flaked sea salt
freshly ground black pepper

Chimichurri sauce
15g bunch of fresh flatleaf parsley
1 long red chilli, deseeded and
    roughly chopped
1 garlic clove, roughly chopped
1 tsp dried oregano
1 tbsp red wine vinegar
1 tbsp cold water
2 tbsp extra virgin olive oil

Onion and radish salad
2 large mild onions
12 small radishes, sliced
handful of cherry tomatoes, halved
15g bunch of fresh coriander
flaked sea salt
freshly ground black pepper

SPICY LAMB STEAKS WITH TABBOULEH

340 calories per portion

This tabbouleh recipe makes enough for six, so keep some aside to enjoy as a healthy salad with cooked chicken, spicy prawns or a few cubes of feta cheese the next day. Alternatively, stick an extra couple of lamb steaks in the marinade and make the whole meal for six instead. Have a dollop of fat-free yoghurt if you like, but add an extra eight calories for each tablespoonful.

Serves 4
Prep: 20 minutes
Cooking time: 10 minutes

4 lean lamb steaks (each
   about 130g)
1 tsp ground cumin
1 tsp ground coriander
2 tbsp fresh lemon juice
1 tbsp harissa paste (or crushed
   red chillies)
½ tsp flaked sea salt
2 tsp sunflower oil, for frying
lemon wedges, for squeezing
freshly ground black pepper

Tabbouleh salad
1 tsp flaked sea salt, plus extra
   to season
200g bulgur wheat
½ cucumber, cut into small chunks
½ medium red onion, finely sliced
200g cherry tomatoes, halved
25g bunch of fresh mint, leaves
   roughly chopped
40g bunch of fresh flatleaf parsley,
   leaves roughly chopped
2 garlic cloves, crushed
2 tbsp fresh lemon juice
freshly ground black pepper

Put the lamb steaks on a board and trim away all the visible fat – don't worry, there will still be plenty within the meat for flavour. Mix the cumin, coriander, lemon juice, harissa in a bowl, then season with the salt and plenty of freshly ground black pepper. Add the lamb steaks and turn until lightly coated. You can leave the lamb to marinate for up to 4 hours at this point if you like.

To make the salad, half fill a medium saucepan with just-boiled water from the kettle, stir in the salt and bring to the boil. Add the bulgur wheat, bring the water back to the boil and cook for 10 minutes or until tender.

Place a large non-stick frying pan over a medium-high heat and brush with a little oil. Alternatively, use a lightly greased griddle pan. Shake the excess marinade off the lamb and cook for 3–5 minutes on each side or until done to taste. Make sure the spices don't burn! Transfer the lamb to a warm plate and let it rest for 5 minutes.

Drain the bulgur wheat well in a sieve under running water until cold. Drain again and tip into a large serving bowl. Add all the other salad ingredients, season with a good pinch of salt and plenty of ground black pepper and toss well together.

Spoon the tabbouleh on to plates and add the hot lamb. Drizzle with any resting juices and serve with lemon wedges for squeezing on top.

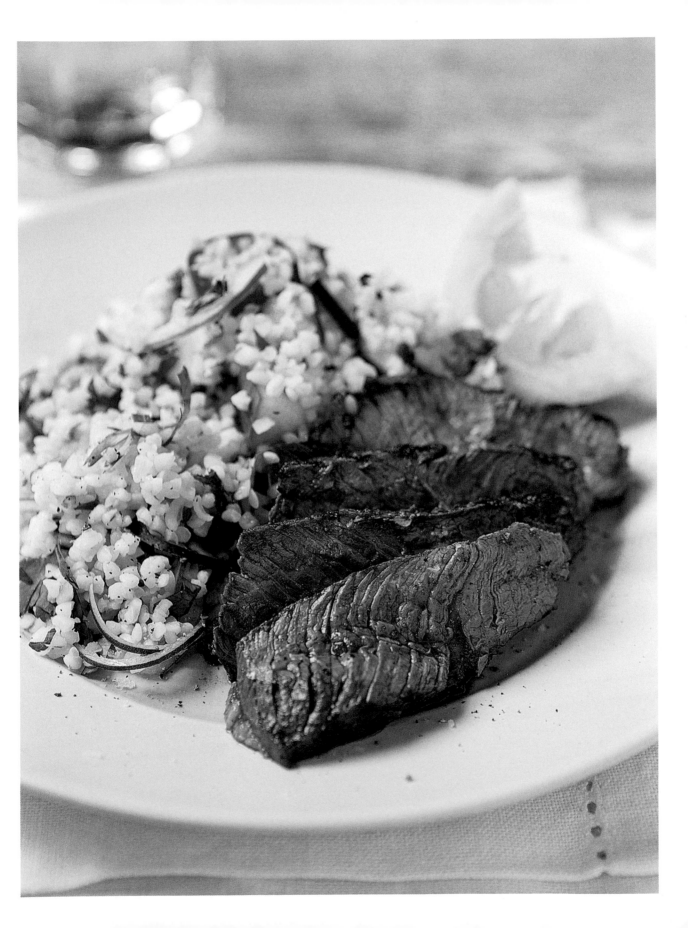

CRISPY PORK SCHNITZEL WITH POTATO SALAD

406 calories per portion

Use wholemeal bread for the breadcrumbs and they'll have enough colour to fool anyone into thinking your schnitzels have been fried, not baked. A couple of medium slices, crusts and all, should make enough crumbs to coat two schnitzels. Team with our special potato salad. Aah, Vienna…

Serves 2
Prep: 20 minutes
Cooking time: 15 minutes

2 pork loin steaks (each about 150g)
oil, for spraying
50g fresh wholemeal breadcrumbs
finely grated zest of ½ small lemon
1 tbsp finely chopped fresh
    thyme leaves
1 tsp paprika
2 tbsp fat-free natural yoghurt
50g watercress, spinach and
    rocket salad
lemon wedges, for squeezing
flaked sea salt
freshly ground black pepper

Potato, celery and apple salad
150g baby new potatoes,
    well scrubbed
2 tbsp light mayonnaise
2 tbsp fat-free natural yoghurt
1 red-skinned eating apple,
    quartered, cored and sliced
2 celery sticks, trimmed and sliced
½ small red onion, finely sliced
flaked sea salt
freshly ground black pepper

To start the potato salad, half fill a small pan with water and bring it to the boil. Add the potatoes, bring the water back to the boil and cook for 15–18 minutes or until they're just tender. Drain, then plunge the potatoes into a bowl of cold water and leave to cool.

While the potatoes are cooking, make the schnitzels. Preheat the oven to 200°C/Fan 180°C/Gas 6. Cut any visible fat off the pork steaks and place each one between 2 sheets of cling film. Bash them with a rolling pin, or the side of a meat mallet, until they're about 1cm thick, trying to keep the shape as even as possible. Remove the cling film and season the pork. Mist a baking tray with oil.

Put the breadcrumbs in a bowl with the lemon zest, thyme, paprika, a good pinch of salt and some black pepper. Mix well, then scatter just a quarter of the flavoured crumbs over a large plate. Put the yoghurt in a bowl.

Take a pork steak and dip it into the yoghurt until lightly coated on both sides. Then place it flat on the breadcrumbs on the plate and top with a quarter more of the crumbs. Press the crumbs on to the pork until evenly covered on both sides. Put the pork on the greased baking tray and prepare the other schnitzel in the same way. Spray the schnitzels with oil and bake them for 12–15 minutes until golden and crisp.

Meanwhile, finish the salad. Mix the mayonnaise and yoghurt in a medium bowl. Cut each of the potatoes in half and toss with the mayonnaise dressing. Add the apple, celery and onion, then stir well and season with salt and pepper to taste.

Divide the potato salad between 2 plates – there's quite a lot, so save some for a packed lunch the next day if you like. Lean a hot pork schnitzel across each heap of potato salad and add the salad leaves. Serve with lemon wedges for squeezing.

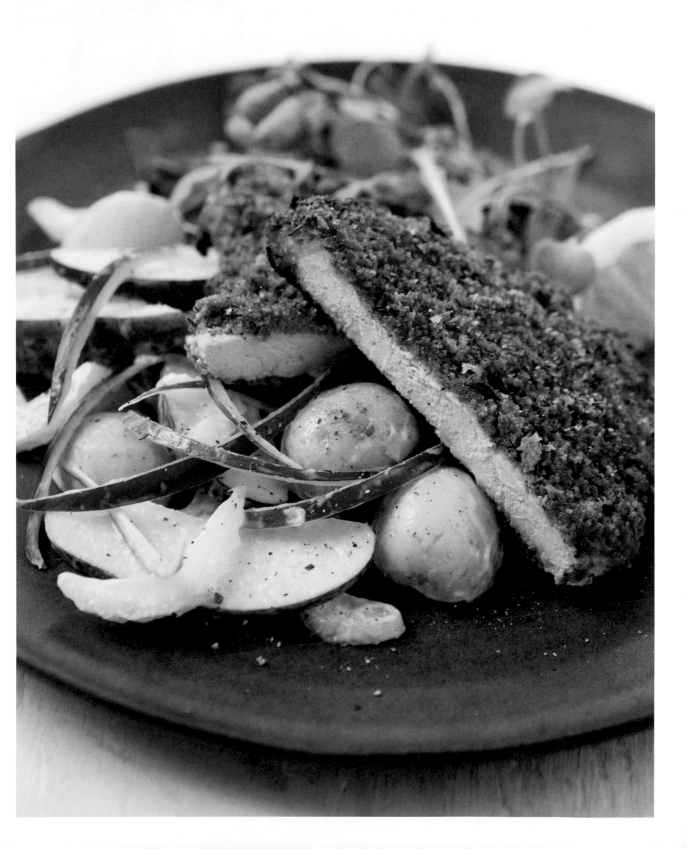

FAMILY
FAVOURITES

"We all need a bit of comfort, and for me and lots of others that means food. And you know what? On our diet you can still have your comfort food. We've come up with warm and scrumptious dishes that all the family will love, including fish pie, chicken and vegetable pot pies – even a proper roast beef dinner for Sunday. And Si now has a lower-cal version of that Geordie comfort classic – pan haggerty. Get stuck in."

Dave

HOME-MADE FISHCAKES

187 calories per portion

Fishcakes are a great standby and everyone loves them. These contain more fish than potato, so they taste even better, are less calorific than most – and there's extra fish for your cakehole! A little tartare sauce goes down a treat, but don't forget to add 15 calories per teaspoon. If you don't like the flavour of smoked fish, just use an extra 100g of cod or haddock.

Serves 4
Prep: 20 minutes
Cooking time: 30–35 minutes

275g potatoes (preferably Maris Pipers), peeled and cut into rough 3cm chunks
300g thick cod or haddock fillet, unskinned
100g smoked haddock fillet, unskinned (preferably undyed)
1 bay leaf
finely grated zest of ½ small lemon
4 spring onions, trimmed and finely sliced (including lots of green)
oil, for spraying
1 large egg
50g fresh wholemeal breadcrumbs
1 tsp paprika
lemon wedges, to serve
flaked sea salt
freshly ground black pepper

Put the potatoes in a pan of cold water and bring to the boil. Reduce the heat slightly and simmer for 15 minutes or until the potatoes are soft but not falling apart.

While the potatoes are cooking, put the fish fillets in a large saucepan, placing the thicker fillets on the bottom of the pan. Cover with cold water and add the bay leaf. Put a tight-fitting lid on the pan and gently bring to a simmer, then immediately take the pan off the heat. Leave the fish to stand for 5 minutes.

Drain the potatoes well in a colander, tip them back into the pan and mash them until smooth or pass them through a potato ricer. Put the mash in a large bowl and season with salt and black pepper.

Drain the fish really well in a colander and break it into large chunks, discarding the skin and any bones as you go. Put the fish in the same bowl as the mashed potato and stir in the lemon zest and spring onions with a large wooden spoon – try not to break up the fish too much. Divide the mixture into 4 balls and flatten each ball to about 3cm thick. If the mixture is too soft to shape into balls, cover and leave it to cool for a while. The potato will stiffen up as it cools. Lightly mist a baking tray with oil.

Beat the egg in a shallow bowl. Mix the breadcrumbs with the paprika in a large bowl. Dip a fishcake into the egg, coating it on all sides. Allow any excess egg to drip off the fishcake and then place it in the breadcrumbs, turning it and pressing firmly to get an even coating of crumbs on all sides. Place the fishcake on the greased tray and prepare the rest in the same way. Leave them to chill in the fridge until you're ready to cook, but use them within 24 hours.

To cook the fishcakes, preheat the oven to 220°C/Fan 200°C/Gas 7. Mist the fishcakes with the oil and bake them for 15–20 minutes until crisp and golden brown. Serve with vegetables or a lightly dressed salad and some lemon wedges for squeezing.

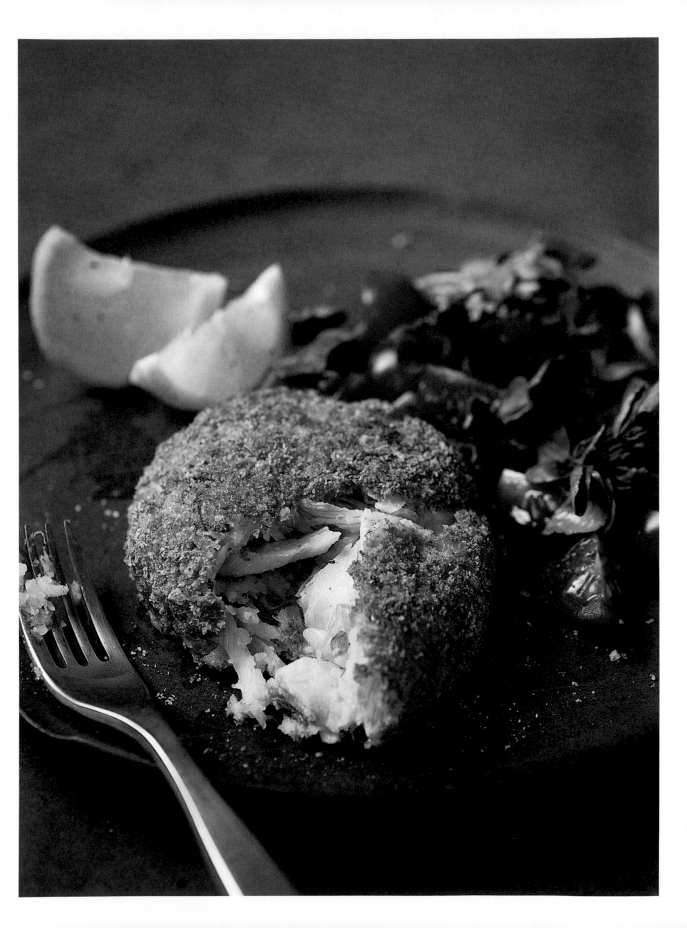

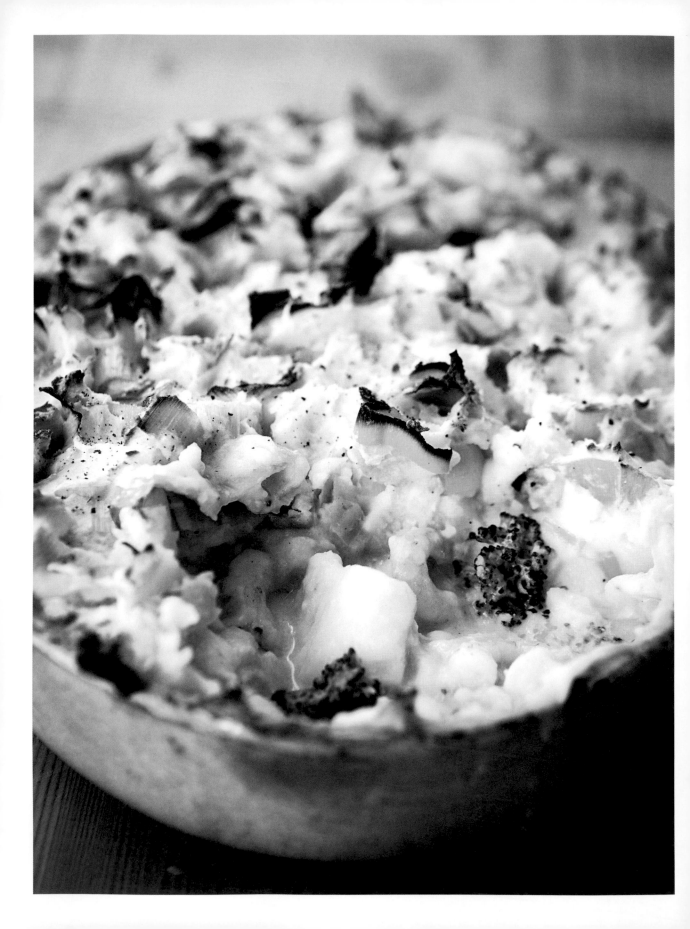

FISHERMAN'S PIE WITH LEEKY MASH

315 calories per portion

You all know we love a fish pie and we've come up with a lighter than usual version, topped with a fab leek-filled mash. Sometimes we make this, sometimes we go back to our full-fat recipe and we're happy because both are great.

To make the leeky mash, peel the potatoes and cut them into rough 4cm chunks. Put the potatoes in a large saucepan and cover them with cold water. Bring the water to the boil, then reduce the heat slightly and simmer for 18–20 minutes or until the potatoes are very tender.

Meanwhile, melt the butter in a non-stick frying pan and fry the leeks for 5 minutes until softened but not coloured, stirring often. Drain the potatoes, then tip them back into the pan and mash with the milk and seasoning to taste until smooth. Stir in the leeks and set aside.

Preheat the oven to 220°C/Fan 200°C/Gas 7. Half fill a medium pan with water and bring it to the boil, then add the broccoli florets and bring the water back to the boil. Cook the broccoli for 2 minutes, then drain it in a sieve under running water until cold. Put to one side.

Cut the white fish fillet and haddock into chunks of about 3cm and set aside. Pour the 400ml of milk into a large non-stick saucepan and bring it to a gentle simmer. Mix the cornflour and water together in a small bowl until smooth, then pour this into the warm milk. Bring to a gentle simmer and cook over a low heat for 2–3 minutes, stirring constantly with a wooden spoon until the sauce is thick and smooth. Season with salt and lots of freshly ground black pepper.

Add the fish pieces to the sauce and cook for 2 minutes, stirring only occasionally so the fish doesn't break up too much. Add the frozen prawns and broccoli to the mixture and stir gently until evenly combined.

Spoon the fish mixture into a 1.5-litre, shallow ovenproof dish. Top with the leeky mash, spooning it around the outside of the dish before working your way into the middle. Place the dish on a baking tray and cook the pie in the oven for 35–40 minutes or until lightly browned, bubbling and hot throughout.

Serves 5
Prep: 20 minutes
Cooking time: 1 hour 10 minutes

---

1 medium head of broccoli, cut into small florets
350g thick white fish fillet, such as cod, skinned
150g smoked haddock (preferably undyed), skinned
400ml semi-skimmed milk
4 tbsp cornflour
4 tbsp cold water
150g cooked, peeled prawns, thawed if frozen
flaked sea salt
freshly ground black pepper

Leeky mash
600g floury potatoes, such as King Edwards or Maris Pipers
20g butter
2 medium leeks, trimmed and cut into 1cm slices
3 tbsp semi-skimmed milk
flaked sea salt
freshly ground black pepper

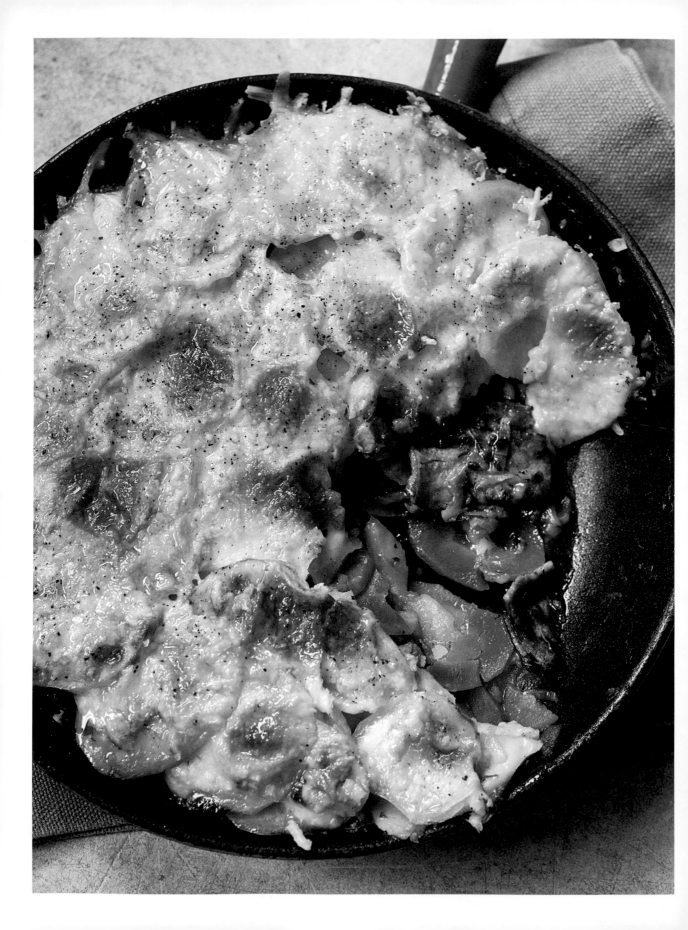

PAN HAGGERTY LITE

320 calories per portion (if serving 4); 213 calories per portion (if serving 6)

One of Si's one-pot wonders, this is a calorie-friendly version of the classic Geordie comfort food. "Hold the butter, use half-fat cheese but still enjoy a well-toned top toon taste, pet, hinny…" (Si). "Oh, do shut up!" (Dave).

Trim any visible fat off the bacon and cut the rashers into 2cm-wide strips. Mist a large shallow casserole dish or a high-sided flameproof frying pan with oil and place it over a medium heat. Add the bacon and onions to the pan and cook for 8–10 minutes, stirring regularly until the onions are softened and beginning to brown. Stir in the parsley, if using, and tip everything on to a plate.

Place half the potatoes in an even layer over the bottom of the pan and top them with a third of the onion and bacon mixture. Add half the carrots, scattering them as evenly as you can, and top with more onion and bacon. Season with lots of black pepper, then add a final layer of carrots and the remaining onion mixture. Top with the rest of the potatoes.

Pour over the chicken stock and cover the pan with a lid or tight-fitting foil. The vegetables on top should be steamed in the hot stock if your lid fits tightly enough.

Bring to a simmer on the hob and leave to cook for about 20 minutes or until the vegetables are tender. You can test them with the tip of a knife. Cook for longer if they remain firm after 20 minutes.

When all the vegetables are soft, but retaining their shape, preheat the grill to its hottest setting. Sprinkle the cheese over the veg and pop the pan under the grill until the cheese is melted and golden. Serve the pan haggerty in bowls with lots of freshly cooked green vegetables or a large salad on the side.

Serves 4–6
Prep: 20 minutes
Cooking time: about 20 minutes

200g rindless lean smoked back bacon rashers

oil, for spraying

2 medium onions, thinly sliced

20g bunch of fresh parsley, leaves finely chopped (optional)

6 medium potatoes (about 675g), peeled and cut into 5mm slices

5 medium carrots, peeled and cut into 5mm slices

500ml hot chicken stock, made with 1 chicken stock cube

100g half-fat mature Cheddar cheese, finely grated

freshly ground black pepper

VEGGIE BEAN BURGERS

237 calories per portion

Well, we all know what pulses can do to you but they're good for the heart and they taste great too. These beany burgers are excellent served warm or cold and they make a welcome addition to a packed lunch, served with a nice crunchy salad and our creamy sauce.

Serves 4
Prep: 20 minutes
Cooking time: 25 minutes

1 tbsp sunflower oil, plus extra for brushing
1 medium onion, roughly chopped
2 garlic cloves, crushed
1 tsp ground cumin
1 tsp ground coriander
finely grated zest of 1 lemon
400g can of chickpeas, drained and rinsed
400g can of red kidney beans, drained and rinsed
50g fresh white breadcrumbs
1 heaped tsp flaked sea salt
lemon wedges, for squeezing
baby gem lettuce, tomato and red onion salad, to serve
freshly ground black pepper

Creamy mango sauce
3 tbsp fat-free natural yoghurt
2 tbsp half-fat crème fraiche
2 tsp mango chutney
½ tsp fresh lemon juice

Heat the oil in a medium non-stick pan and gently fry the onion and garlic for 5 minutes until softened, stirring regularly. Stir in the cumin, coriander and lemon zest and cook for 1 minute more, while stirring. Leave to cool for 5 minutes. Preheat the oven to 210°C/ Fan 190°C/Gas 6½.

Tip the spicy onions into a food processor, add the chickpeas, kidney beans, breadcrumbs, salt and lots of black pepper. Blitz until well combined but not smooth. You want the mixture to have some texture and show small pieces of the beans but to be puréed enough to hold together when rolled. You may need to remove the lid and push the mixture down a couple of times with a rubber spatula until the right consistency is reached. (If there's not enough room in your food processor for all the mixture, blend it in 2 batches.)

Tip the mixture into a bowl and adjust the seasoning to taste, then divide it into 8 portions. Roll each portion into a ball and flatten it into a burger shape, just over 1.5cm thick. Place the burgers on a baking tray lightly brushed with oil, then brush them with a little more oil and bake in the oven for 10 minutes.

Take the tray out of the oven and gently turn the burgers over with a spatula. Put them back in the oven for another 10 minutes until they're lovely and golden and crunchy on the outside.

While the burgers are cooking, make the sauce. Mix the yoghurt, crème fraiche, mango chutney and lemon juice in a small bowl until combined.

Serve 2 burgers per person, topped with a little of the mango sauce, a colourful salad on the side and some lemon wedges for squeezing. Keep any leftover burgers in the fridge and use them within a couple of days. You can give them a quick blast in the microwave to take off the chill.

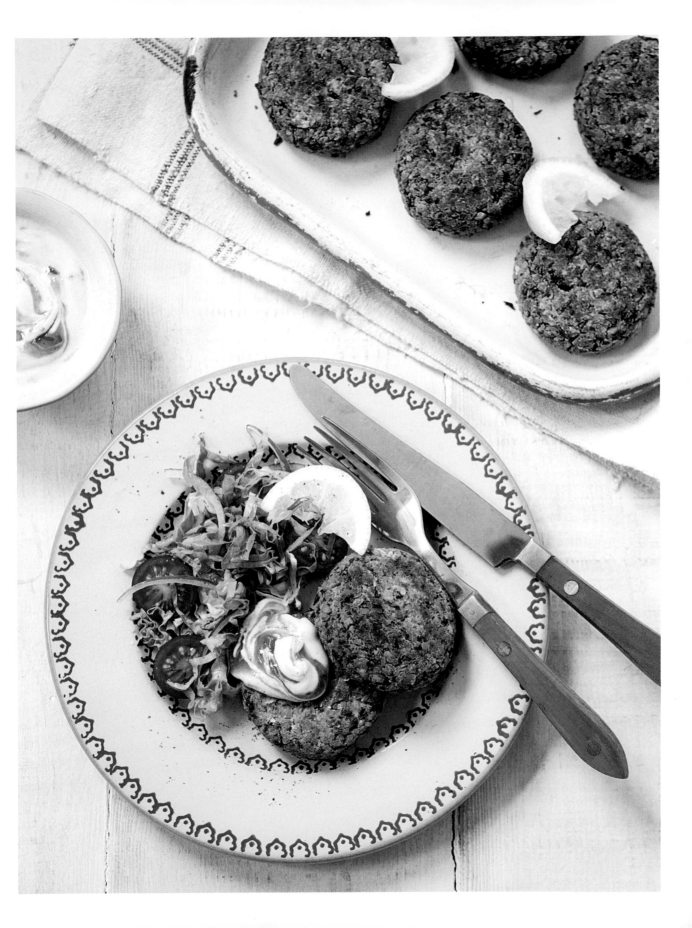

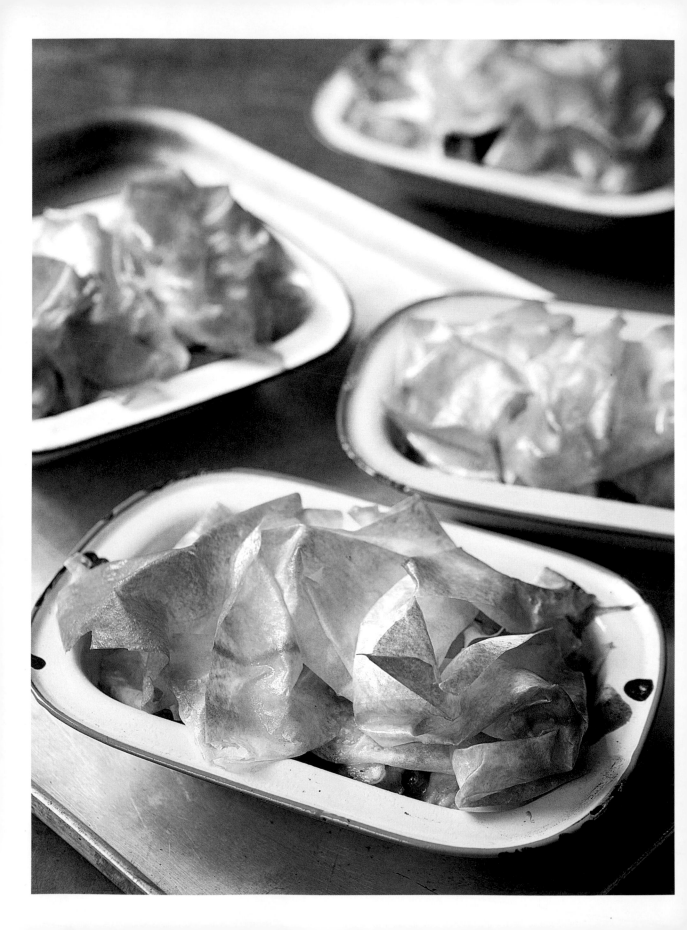

SPEEDY CHICKEN AND VEGETABLE POT PIES

267 calories per portion

We could never give up our pies and these little beauties are ready in no time. They're a great way to use up any lean cooked chicken you have left over from a Sunday roast too. Add a splash of white wine to the sauce if you like – a tablespoon will bring an additional 12 calories to the recipe.

Preheat the oven to 220°C/Fan 200°C/Gas 7. Trim any visible fat off the bacon rashers and cut them into strips about 1.5cm wide. Mist a large non-stick saucepan with oil and place it over a medium heat. Add the bacon to the pan, then stir in the mushrooms and cook for 4 minutes, stirring regularly until they are beginning to brown.

Add the leek and chicken and cook for 1 minute more, stirring. Sprinkle over the flour and cook for a few seconds before gradually adding the stock, just a little at a time.

Bring to a simmer and season well with a pinch of salt and lots of freshly ground black pepper. Add the broccoli florets and peas and bring the water back to a simmer. Cook for 4 minutes, while stirring, until the sauce thickens, then remove from the heat and stir in the crème fraiche.

Divide the mixture between 4 individual pie dishes – each will need to hold about 350ml. Spray each sheet of filo pastry with oil and cut them into 4 wide strips. Working quickly, top each dish with 3 strips of the filo, oiled-side up, crumpling and scrunching them loosely as you go.

Place the dishes on a baking tray and bake the pies in the centre of the oven for 12–15 minutes or until the pastry is golden brown and the filling is hot and bubbling.

Serves 4
Prep: 10 minutes
Cooking time: 24 minutes

---

2 rindless lean smoked back
    bacon rashers
oil, for spraying
150g button mushrooms, wiped
    and halved
1 slender leek, trimmed and
    finely sliced
2 skinless boneless roast chicken
    breasts, cut into small pieces
    (about 200g), or lean leftover
    roast chicken
25g plain flour
500ml chicken stock, made with
    1 stock cube
150g broccoli, cut into small florets
75g frozen peas
2 tbsp half-fat crème fraiche
3 sheets of filo pastry, each
    about 45g
flaked sea salt
freshly ground black pepper

EASY CHICKEN BAKE

395 calories per portion

This colourful one-pan supper is dead easy to make and tastes luxuriously good. It's already a firm favourite with our families. Once you've got all your veg prepared and the chicken stuffed, you can leave it to bake while you get on with something else.

Serves 4
Prep time: 20 minutes
Cooking time: 35 minutes

3 medium courgettes
25g extra-mature Cheddar cheese
45g sun-dried tomatoes, well
   drained (about 6 pieces)
4 boneless, skinless chicken breasts
   (each about 175g)
1 medium red onion, cut into
   12 wedges
2 medium sweet potatoes (each
   about 225g), peeled and cut into
   3cm chunks
2 yellow peppers, deseeded and cut
   into 3cm chunks
1 tbsp extra virgin olive oil
½ tsp dried chilli flakes (optional)
12 cherry vine tomatoes
flaked sea salt
freshly ground black pepper

Preheat the oven to 220°C/Fan 200°C/Gas 7. Trim the courgettes and cut 2 of them into diagonal slices, about 1.5cm thick. Grate the third courgette on the medium-fine side of your grater, not too fine or too coarse if possible. You want it to be in fairly thin strands.

Scoop up the grated courgette in your hands and squeeze out as much water as you can, then put it in a bowl.

Grate the cheese on the medium-fine setting of your grater – the same as the courgette – and add it to the courgette. Cut the sun-dried tomatoes into rough 1cm chunks and add them to the bowl. Season with a pinch of salt and some freshly ground black pepper, then mix well.

Put the chicken breasts on a board and cut a 10cm slit in each one, horizontally. Cut almost all the way through so you can open the chicken breast like a book. Divide the grated courgette mixture between the chicken breasts and close the 2 sides to hold the filling. This stuffing will help keep the chicken deliciously moist as it cooks.

Put the sliced courgettes in a large roasting tin and add the red onion wedges, sweet potatoes and yellow peppers. Drizzle over the oil, season with salt and lots of freshly ground black pepper and toss together well.

Nestle the stuffed chicken breasts among the vegetables, season with ground black pepper and sprinkle with the chilli flakes, if using. Bake for 25 minutes.

Remove the pan from the oven and scatter in the cherry tomatoes. Put it back in the oven for another 10 minutes or until the chicken is cooked and the vegetables are tender and lightly browned.

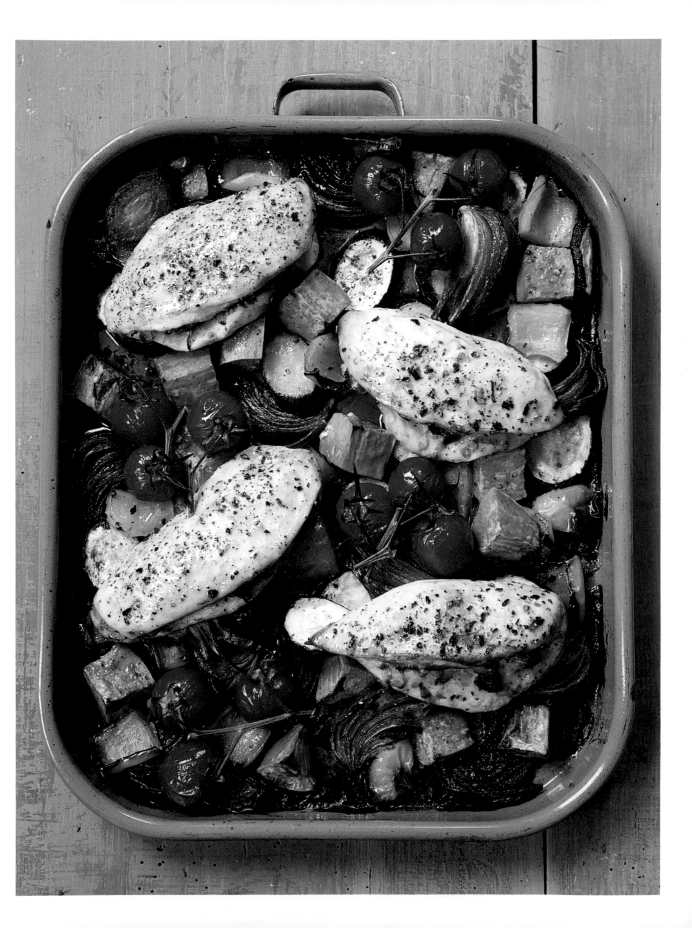

LIVER AND BACON WITH ONION GRAVY

254 calories per portion

A good plate of liver and bacon has always been one of our very favourite meals so we're dead chuffed that we can still enjoy it. Serve with lots of greens and a smidgen of mash (see pages 180–181).

Serves 4
Prep: 10 minutes
Cooking time: about 15 minutes

450g lambs' or calves' liver, sliced
  (thawed, if frozen)
4 tsp plain flour
20g butter
1 tsp sunflower oil
1 medium onion, fairly thinly sliced
2 rindless lean back bacon rashers
  (about 55g), each cut into 2cm-
  wide strips
500ml beef stock, made with
  1 stock cube
2 tsp tomato ketchup
flaked sea salt
freshly ground black pepper

Rinse the liver in a colander under cold water and drain it well on kitchen paper. Put 2 teaspoons of the flour in a large bowl and season with plenty of salt and pepper. Add the liver to the bowl and turn it in the flour until lightly coated.

Melt half the butter with the oil in a large non-stick frying pan over a medium heat. Tap the excess flour off each slice of liver and add them to the pan using tongs. Cook for 1½–2 minutes on each side until lightly browned but not completely cooked through, then pop them on to a plate.

Turn down the heat and melt the remaining butter in the same pan. Add the sliced onion and cook for a minute or so, stirring to separate the layers. Next, add the bacon and cook together for another 5 minutes or until the onion is softened and pale golden brown, stirring often.

Sprinkle the remaining flour over the onion and bacon and cook for a few seconds, stirring. Pour the hot stock slowly into the pan, stirring constantly. Bring to a simmer, stir in the ketchup and cook over a medium heat until the gravy is thickened and glossy.

Put the liver back in the pan and heat it through in the onion gravy for 2–3 minutes until hot, stirring. Season to taste with salt and pepper. Serve the liver and bacon with a small portion of mashed potatoes and lots of freshly cooked greens.

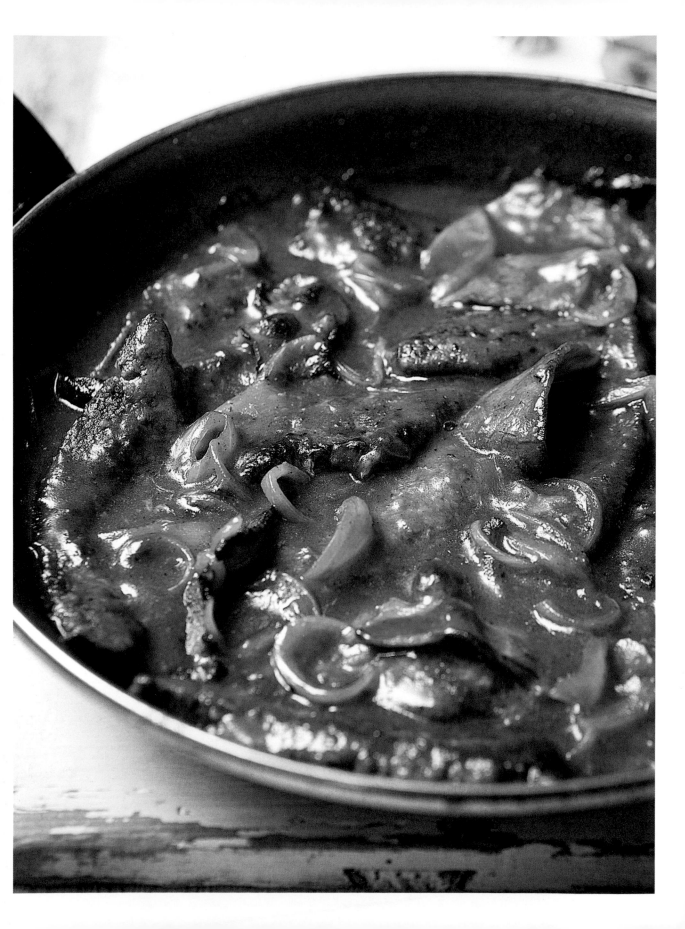

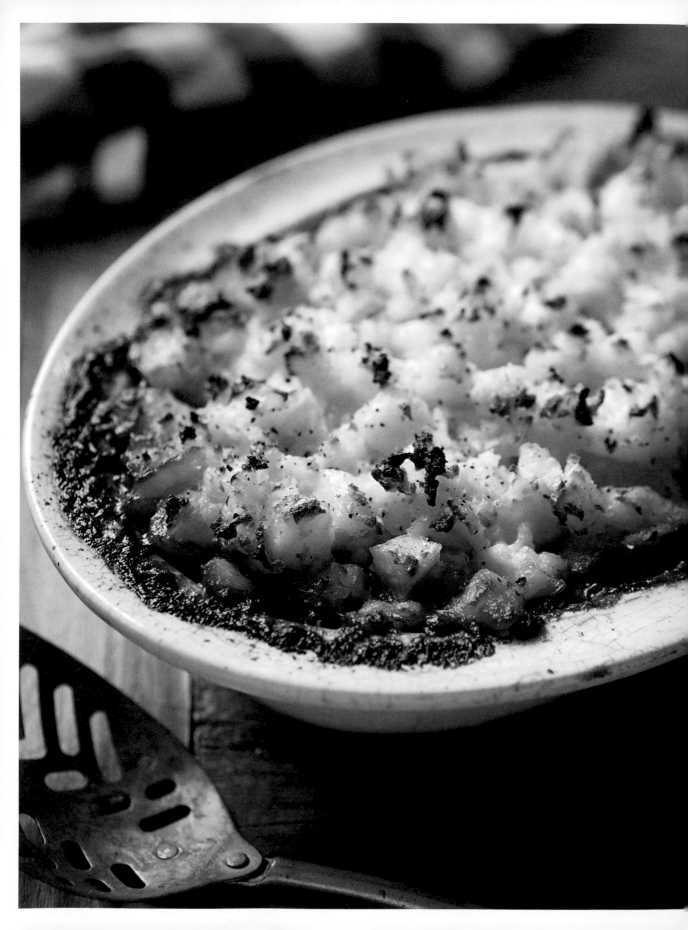

MINCE AND VEGETABLE PIE
WITH TUMBLED SPUDS

366 calories per portion (if serving 4); 292 calories per portion (if serving 5)

A good old meat and potato pie is always a welcome sight. This one is made with extra-lean beef to keep the calories down but there's plenty of flavour. And, if you like, you could top this pie with mashed sweet potatoes instead of the regular sort.

Place a large non-stick saucepan or flameproof casserole dish over a medium heat and cook the mince with the onion, leeks and carrots for 5 minutes until lightly coloured. Break up the meat with a couple of wooden spoons as it cooks.

Stir in the flour and cook for a few seconds, stirring. Add the tomato purée, beef stock, herbs and Worcestershire sauce, then season with a good pinch of salt and plenty of freshly ground black pepper. Bring the mixture to a simmer and cook without covering for 20 minutes, stirring occasionally.

Meanwhile, preheat the oven to 220°C/Fan 200°C/Gas 7. Half fill a large saucepan with water and bring it to the boil. Peel the potatoes and cut them into rough 2cm chunks. Add the potatoes to the boiling water, bring it back to the boil and cook for 5 minutes. Remove the pan from the heat and drain the potatoes in a colander. Tip them back into the saucepan, add the butter and lots of seasoning, then bash or lightly mash the potatoes.

Pour the beef mixture into a 1.8-litre, shallow ovenproof dish. Tumble the potatoes on top and season with lots of ground black pepper. Bake for 25–30 minutes until the topping is golden and the filling is bubbling.

Serves 4–5
Prep: 15 minutes
Cooking time: 40–50 minutes

500g extra-lean minced beef
1 medium onion, chopped
2 slender leeks, trimmed and sliced
2 medium carrots, peeled and diced
2 tbsp plain flour
2 tbsp tomato purée
500ml beef stock, made with 1 beef
    stock cube (Oxo is good)
1½ tsp dried mixed herbs
1 tbsp Worcestershire sauce
flaked sea salt
freshly ground black pepper

Potato topping
600g medium potatoes, preferably
    Maris Pipers
15g butter
flaked sea salt
freshly ground black pepper

ONE-PAN LAMB ROAST WITH GRAVY

378 calories per portion

The easiest roast lamb dinner you'll ever make – and it's lower in calories than usual too. You don't have to make the red wine gravy, but we think it makes the whole meal that bit more special. You can use lamb cutlets or, if you prefer, a couple of French-trimmed lamb racks separated into cutlets. They are more pricy but you'll save time trimming the fat.

Serves 4
Prep: 25 minutes
Cooking time: 50 minutes

500g baby new potatoes, well
   washed and cut in half
2 large carrots, (about 350g in all),
   peeled and cut into 2.5cm chunks
2 medium parsnips, (about 350g
   in all) peeled and cut into
   2.5cm chunks
1 medium onion, cut into
   12 wedges
1 tbsp olive oil
1 tbsp roughly chopped fresh thyme
   leaves or 1 tsp dried thyme
1 tbsp finely chopped fresh rosemary
   leaves or 1 tsp dried rosemary
8 well-trimmed lamb cutlets
3 small courgettes
2 tbsp ready-made mint sauce
300ml lamb stock, made with
   ½ lamb stock cube
100ml red wine
good pinch of caster sugar
2 tsp cornflour
2 tbsp cold water
flaked sea salt
freshly ground black pepper

Preheat the oven to 200°C/Fan 180°C/Gas 6. Put the potatoes, carrots, parsnips, onion and olive oil in your largest baking tray or grill pan – you want it to be fairly shallow so a roasting tin isn't ideal. The pan will need to go on the hob a bit later, so make sure it's a sturdy one. Sprinkle over the thyme and rosemary and season with salt and pepper. Toss all the vegetables together and roast for 20 minutes.

While the vegetables are cooking, carefully trim any visible fat off the lamb with a sharp knife. This may take a little while but is worth it to reduce the total fat and calorie content of your meal. Season the lamb on both sides with salt and pepper. Trim the courgettes and cut them into diagonal slices of about 1.5cm thick.

Take the baking tray out of the oven and scatter the courgettes over the other vegetables. Nestle the lamb cutlets among the vegetables and drizzle with the mint sauce. Put the tray back in the oven for 25 minutes or until all the vegetables are tender and the lamb is lightly browned.

Transfer the vegetables and lamb to a warmed serving platter and cover with foil to help keep them hot while you make the gravy. Place the baking tray over a medium heat and add the stock, wine and a good pinch of sugar. Bring to a simmer. Cook for 2 minutes, stirring to lift any tasty brown bits from the bottom of the pan.

Mix the cornflour with the water to form a smooth paste and stir this into the stock. Simmer for 2 minutes, stirring constantly. Very carefully pour the gravy into a warmed, wide jug and serve with the lamb.

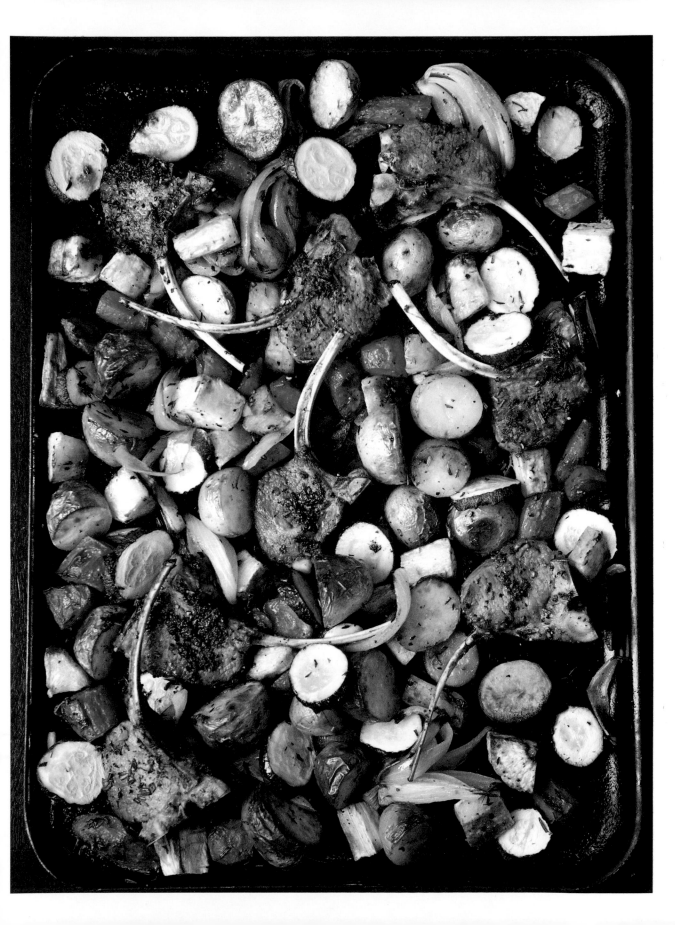

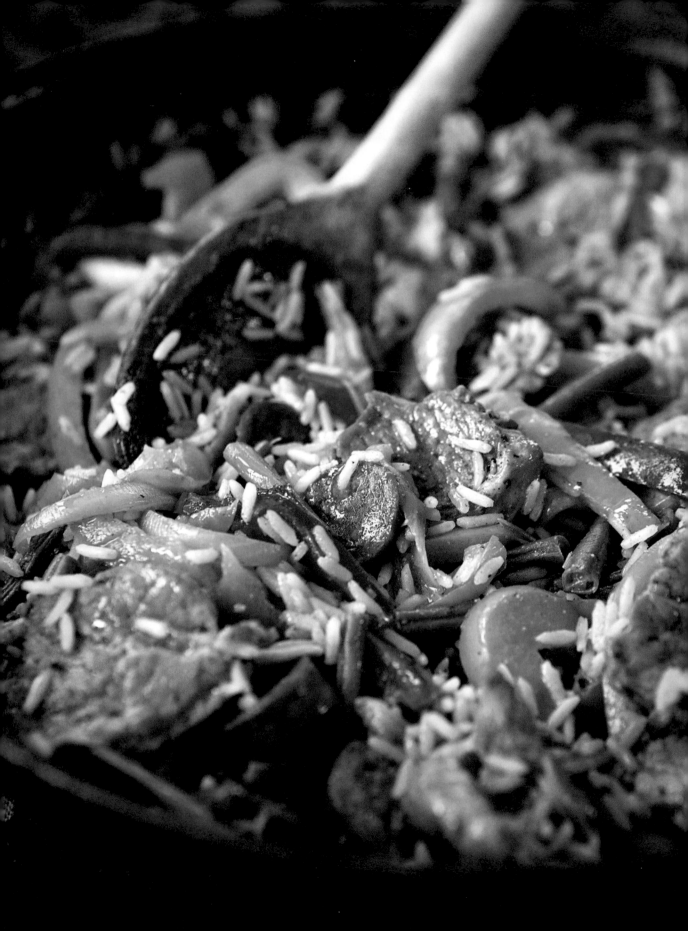

ALL-IN-ONE SPICY PORK AND RICE

395 calories per portion

Lean, tender pork with spicy rice and lots of veggies – what more could you want? This is a scrumptiously simple family supper with big flavours that fulfils all your needs. Only problem is stopping yourself eating too much of it!

Heat the oil in a large, non-stick deep frying pan or sauté pan. Fry the onion wedges over a medium-high heat for 3 minutes until they're softened and lightly browned, stirring regularly.

Season the pork with salt and black pepper, then add it to the pan and stir-fry with the onion for 2 minutes until lightly browned. Add the chorizo, garlic, peppers and beans and stir-fry together for 2 minutes more. Sprinkle with the spices and stir in the rice, then pour over the stock and bring to the boil.

Reduce the heat to a simmer and cook for 20 minutes, stirring regularly, until the liquid has been absorbed and the rice and pork are both lovely and tender.

Serves 4
Prep: 15 minutes
Cooking time: about 30 minutes

2 tsp olive oil
1 medium onion, sliced into
  thin wedges
500g pork tenderloin, trimmed and
  cut into 1cm slices
50g chorizo sausage, skinned and
  cut into 5mm slices
2 garlic cloves, thinly sliced
1 red and 1 orange pepper, deseeded
  and sliced
100g green beans, trimmed and cut
  into short lengths
1 tsp ground cumin
1 tsp ground coriander
½ tsp hot chilli powder
150g easy-cook long-grain rice
750ml chicken stock, made with
  1 stock cube
flaked sea salt
freshly ground black pepper

ROAST BEEF AND GRAVY

480 calories per portion (including potatoes, gravy, squash and Yorkshires)

A Sunday roast with all the trimmings – you can't do without it. This is a real family favourite but we make it fit the diet bill with a few clever little variations.

Serves 6
Prep: 20 minutes
Cooking time: 1 hour and 20 minutes

20g bunch of fresh thyme, leaves very finely chopped
1 tbsp English mustard powder
1.2kg lean rolled beef topside joint
oil, for spraying
6 medium-sized long shallots, trimmed and halved lengthways
100ml red wine, plus 2 tbsp
500ml beef stock, made with 1 stock cube
1½ tbsp gravy powder
3 tbsp cold water
flaked sea salt
freshly ground black pepper

Side dishes
900g medium potatoes, preferably Maris Pipers, peeled and cut into 5cm chunks
oil, for spraying
600g butternut squash, peeled, deseeded and cut into 5cm chunks
6 frozen ready-made Yorkshire puddings (about 50 calories each), cooked according to the packet instructions
freshly cooked carrots and shredded Savoy cabbage, to serve

Preheat the oven to 200°C/Fan 180°C/Gas 6. Mix the thyme, mustard powder, a good pinch of salt and plenty of ground black pepper in a bowl. Spray the beef lightly with the oil and roll it in the herb mixture until lightly coated.

Mist a large non-stick frying pan with oil and place it over a medium-high heat. Add the beef to the pan and brown for 8–10 minutes, turning it every now and then until well coloured on all sides. Put the halved shallots in a sturdy roasting tin and place the beef on top.

To cook the potatoes, half fill a medium pan with water and bring it to the boil. Gently add the potatoes and parboil them for 5 minutes, then drain in a colander and shake them around a bit to roughen up the sides. Spritz with oil and season with salt and pepper, then scatter them on a baking tray. Add the butternut squash and spritz all the vegetables lightly with the oil.

Put the beef and vegetables in the oven, with the beef on the shelf above the potatoes and squash. Roast together for 45 minutes, turning the vegetables halfway through the cooking time. (Add 15 minutes to the cooking time for medium beef and 25 minutes to the cooking time for well-cooked beef.) Remove the beef from the oven and place it on a board, cover loosely with foil, and leave it to rest for 15 minutes. Transfer the shallots to a small baking tray and keep them warm. Cook the potatoes and squash for 15 minutes longer.

Place the beef roasting tin on the hob. Add the 100ml of red wine, then the beef stock and bring to a simmer, stirring to lift the tasty juices from the bottom of the pan. Mix the gravy powder with the water until smooth and stir it into the wine and stock. Bring to a simmer, stirring constantly. Season to taste with salt and lots of black pepper, then stir in the rest of the wine and return to a simmer.

Strain the gravy through a fine sieve into a warmed jug. Carve the beef into thin slices and tip any of the carving and resting juices into the gravy. Serve the beef, Yorkshire puddings, potatoes and squash with gravy and some freshly cooked carrots and cabbage.

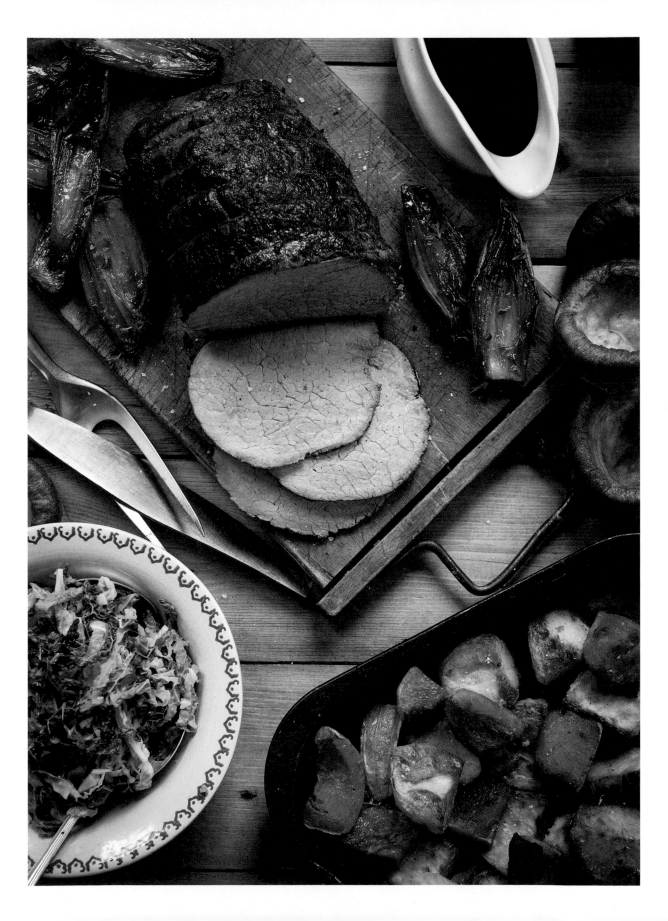

MEALS
WITH MATES

"Tell you what – say nought and they won't even know they're eating diet food. Watch your friends tuck in to chicken Provençal, beef in red wine or stroganoff and you'll have a little smile on your face, smug in the knowledge that you're doing them a bit of good. Tell them afterwards they've just eaten a low-cal meal and they won't believe you! Seriously though, we both love cooking meals for friends and it's not something we'd ever want to stop doing. If we can party without smashing the diet too much, we're happy."

Si

TUNA WITH RATATOUILLE

404 calories per portion

Tuna is a tasty, satisfying fish and makes a really special summery meal when teamed with some delicious Mediterranean ratatouille. Your friends will catch on to this fishy feast…sorry! Buy good-quality tuna so you can eat it rare.

Serves 4
Prep: 20 minutes
Cooking time: about 1 hour and 15 minutes

4 x 200g fresh tuna steaks
1 tsp olive oil
flaked sea salt
freshly ground black pepper

Ratatouille
1 medium aubergine, cut into
    rough 2cm chunks
2 medium courgettes, halved
    lengthways and cut into
    2cm slices
1 large red pepper, deseeded and
    cut into rough 2cm chunks
1 large yellow pepper, deseeded
    and cut into rough 2cm chunks
2 tbsp olive oil
2 small onions, halved and
    finely sliced
4 garlic cloves, finely sliced
1 tsp coriander seeds, lightly crushed
400g can of chopped tomatoes
handful of fresh basil leaves, roughly
    torn, plus extra to garnish
lemon wedges, to serve (optional)
flaked sea salt
freshly ground black pepper

Put the aubergine, courgettes and peppers in a large bowl and toss them with 1 tablespoon of the olive oil until lightly coated. Season with salt and lots of black pepper.

Place a large non-stick frying pan over a high heat and fry the aubergine, courgettes and peppers in 3 batches until lightly browned but not cooked through, turning often. Each batch should only take 2 minutes if the pan is hot enough. Tip each batch into a bowl as soon as it has browned.

Preheat the oven to 190°C/Fan 170°C/Gas 5. Place a flameproof casserole dish over a medium heat – a fairly shallow casserole or ovenproof sauté pan is ideal. Add the remaining oil and fry the onions for 3 minutes, stirring regularly, then add the garlic and coriander seeds and cook for 2 minutes more.

Stir in the tomatoes, then add the lightly browned vegetables and heat through for a couple of minutes. Cover with a lid and cook in the oven for 25–30 minutes. Take the dish out of the oven and stir everything well, then put it back for another 10–15 minutes until the vegetables are soft and the sauce is thick.

When the ratatouille is ready, take it out of the oven and season to taste, then leave it to stand for 10 minutes while you prepare the tuna. Ratatouille tastes much better after it has cooled for a while.

Season the tuna steaks on both sides with salt and lots of coarsely ground black pepper. Brush a large non-stick frying pan or griddle pan with the teaspoon of oil and place it over a high heat.

Cook the tuna for 1½–2½ minutes on each side until done to your taste. Stir the basil leaves into the ratatouille and divide it between 4 plates. Add a tuna steak to each plate and garnish with more basil and lemon wedges if you like.

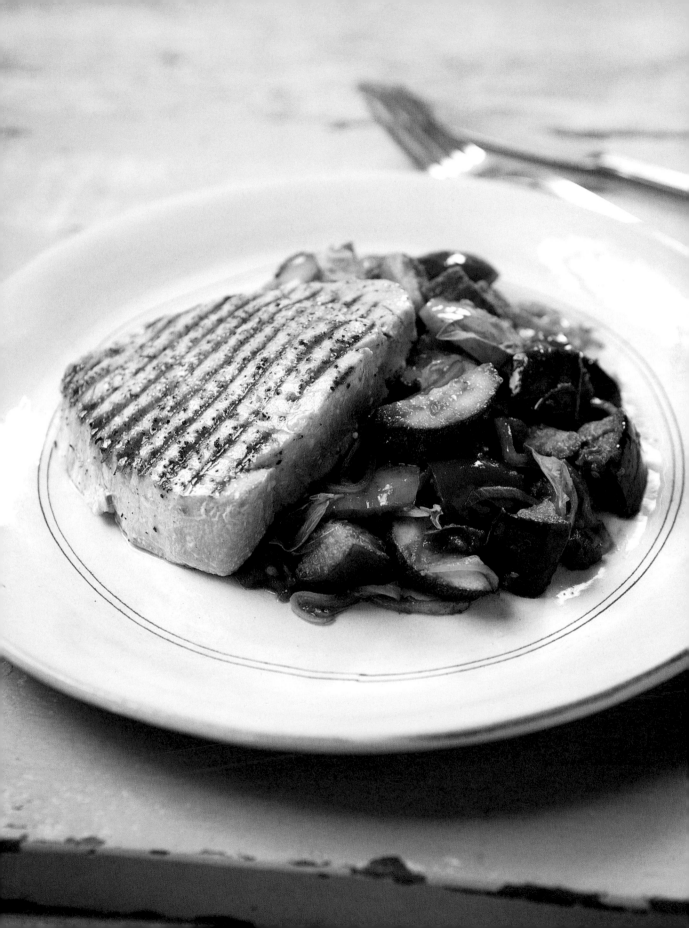

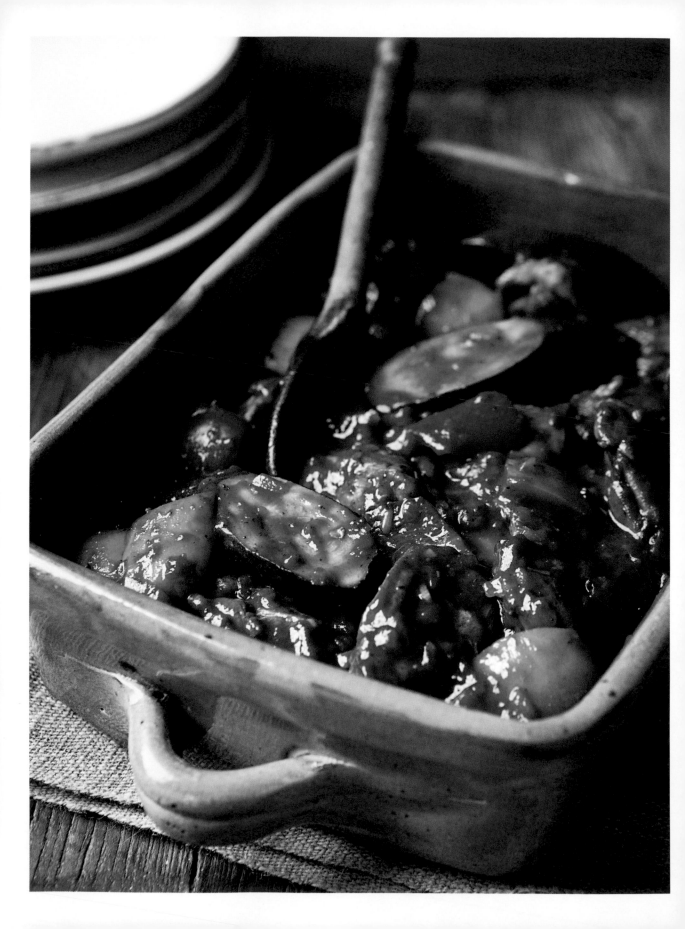

CHICKEN PROVENÇAL

282 calories per portion

Rich in wine and garlic, this is a dish for a party. Put your beret on, imagine yourself on a sunlit balcony in the South of France and enjoy. Oh là là.

Trim all the visible fat off the chicken and cut each thigh in half. Trimming off the fat like this may take a few minutes but will save lots of calories so don't be tempted to skip this step. Use kitchen scissors if you like. Season the chicken with salt and lots of freshly ground black pepper.

Heat the oil in a large non-stick saucepan or flameproof casserole dish. Add the chicken and fry it over a medium-high heat for 2–3 minutes, turning occasionally until lightly coloured. Add the onions, garlic, tomatoes, tomato purée, sugar, stock, herbs and wine to the pan and stir well.

Bring the liquid to a gentle simmer on the hob and cook for 10 minutes, stirring occasionally. Add the peppers and courgettes to the pan, stir well and bring back to a simmer. Cover loosely with a lid and continue to simmer gently for 20 minutes more until the chicken is tender and cooked through, with no pinkness remaining.

Mix the cornflour with the tablespoon of water until smooth. Stir this mixture into the pan and simmer for 1–2 minutes until the sauce has thickened. Serve the chicken just as it is in deep bowls or with a small portion of rice (see pages 178–179).

Serves 6
Prep: 15 minutes
Cooking time: 35–40 minutes

12 boneless, skinless chicken thighs
2 tsp sunflower oil
2 medium onions, thinly sliced
2 garlic cloves, crushed
400g can of chopped tomatoes
2 tbsp tomato purée
1 tsp caster sugar
300ml chicken stock, made with
    1 stock cube
2 heaped tsp dried herbes
    de Provence
100ml red wine
1 large red pepper, deseeded and cut
    into 3cm chunks
1 large yellow pepper, deseeded and
    cut into 3cm chunks
2 medium courgettes, trimmed and
    cut into 2cm slices
1 tbsp cornflour
1 tbsp cold water
flaked sea salt
freshly ground black pepper

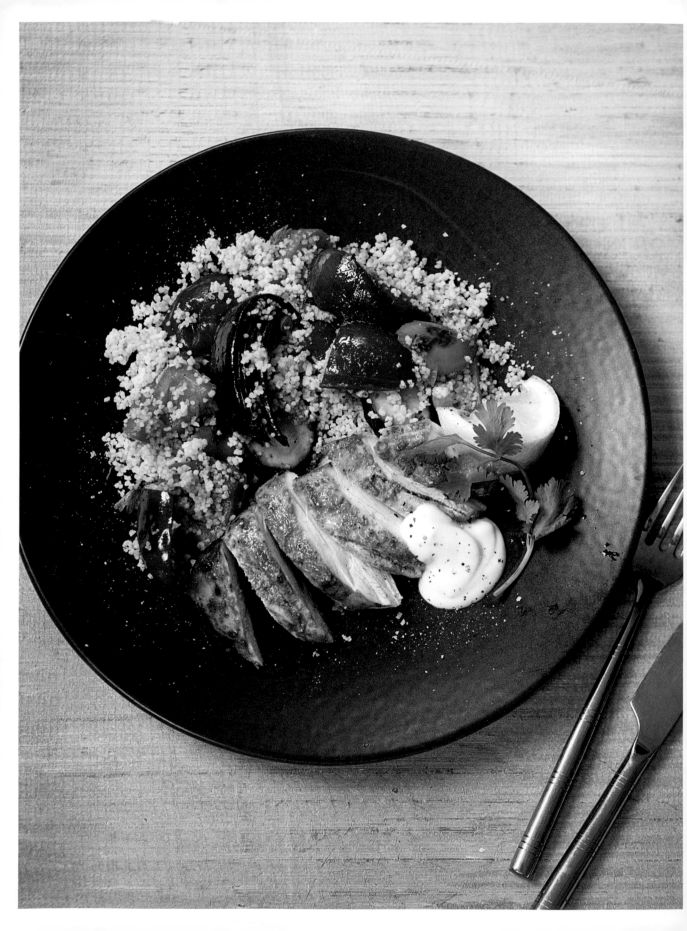

MOROCCAN-STYLE CHICKEN WITH VEGETABLE COUSCOUS

305 calories per portion

We both love sunny Moroccan flavours and spicy harissa paste, as used in this marinade, really is a dieter's friend. It's a great way to add punch without paunch!

To make the marinade, mix the cumin, coriander, harissa, honey, yoghurt, garlic, salt and lots of black pepper in a large bowl. Using a sharp knife, slash each chicken breast diagonally 3 times. Add the chicken breasts to the bowl and coat them well with the marinade, then cover with cling film and chill for 30 minutes.

Deseed the peppers and cut them into 3cm chunks. Cut the onions into 12 wedges. Trim the courgettes and cut them diagonally into 1.5cm slices. Put the vegetables in a bowl and spritz with the oil, then toss them with the chilli flakes, a pinch of sea salt and plenty of freshly ground black pepper.

Preheat the oven to 200°C/Fan 180°C/Gas 6. Place the chicken breasts on a baking tray, slashed-side up. Bake them in the oven for 18–20 minutes or until the chicken is tender and cooked through – there should be no pinkness remaining.

While the chicken is cooking, heat a large non-stick frying pan or wok and add the vegetables. Fry them over a medium-high heat for about 10 minutes or until they are tender and lightly browned, stirring regularly.

Just before the vegetables and chicken are ready, put the couscous in your largest bowl and pour over the hot chicken stock. Cover and leave to stand for 5 minutes. Scatter the coriander over the couscous and toss together with a couple of forks. Add the hot vegetables and mix thoroughly.

Divide the vegetable couscous between 6 warmed plates and add the chicken. Drizzle over any juices. Garnish with coriander sprigs and serve with yoghurt and lemon wedges for squeezing.

Serves 6
Prep: 20 minutes
Cooking time: 18–20 minutes

6 boneless, skinless chicken breasts
   (each about 150g)
1 red pepper
1 yellow pepper
1 orange or green pepper
2 medium red onions
2 medium courgettes
oil, for spraying
1 tsp dried chilli flakes
200g couscous
300ml hot chicken stock, made
   with ½ stock cube
15g bunch of fresh coriander, leaves
   chopped, plus extra to garnish
6 heaped tbsp low-fat natural
   yoghurt
lemon wedges, to serve
flaked sea salt
freshly ground black pepper

Marinade
2 tsp ground cumin
2 tsp ground coriander
1 tsp harissa paste
1 tbsp runny honey
2 tbsp low-fat natural yoghurt
2 garlic cloves, crushed
1 tsp flaked sea salt
freshly ground black pepper

MEATLOAF WITH SPICY TOMATO SAUCE

343 calories per portion

Eat our meatloaf and you won't end up looking like Meatloaf – we take the fat out of hell! We're massive chilli fans, so use fewer chilli flakes in the spicy tomato sauce if you prefer a milder flavour.

Serves 6
Prep: 20 minutes
Cooking time: 50 minutes

1 tsp sunflower oil
1 medium onion, finely chopped
1 medium carrot, peeled and diced
1 celery stick, trimmed and diced
2 garlic cloves, crushed
1 tsp dried thyme
400g lean minced beef (10% fat)
400g lean minced pork (8% fat)
3 tbsp tomato ketchup
1 tbsp Worcestershire sauce
75g fresh white breadcrumbs
20g bunch of flatleaf parsley,
    leaves finely chopped, plus
    extra to garnish
1 medium egg, beaten
1 tsp flaked sea salt
freshly ground black pepper

Spicy tomato sauce
1 tsp sunflower oil
1 medium onion, finely chopped
1 garlic clove, crushed
1 tsp dried chilli flakes
400g can of chopped tomatoes
200ml cold water
1 tsp dried oregano
1 tbsp tomato ketchup

Heat the oil in a medium non-stick saucepan and add the onion, carrot, celery and garlic. Put a lid on the pan and cook for 8 minutes until the veg are well softened, stirring occasionally.

Stir the thyme into the pan and cook with the vegetables for another 2 minutes, stirring constantly. Remove the pan from the heat, tip the contents into a large mixing bowl and leave to cool for 5 minutes. Preheat the oven to 190°C/Fan 170°C/Gas 5. Line the base of a 900g loaf tin with baking parchment.

Add the beef, pork, ketchup, Worcestershire sauce, breadcrumbs, parsley, egg, salt and plenty of black pepper to the bowl with the vegetables and mix well until thoroughly combined. The mixture should feel fairly stiff but moist.

Spoon the mixture into the prepared tin and bake in the centre of the oven for 40 minutes until lightly browned and firm. The internal temperature of the meatloaf should be at least 75°C, so you can check if you have a digital food thermometer handy.

While the meatloaf is cooking, you can make the sauce. Heat the oil in a medium non-stick pan and add the onion and garlic. Cover the pan with a lid and fry gently for 6–8 minutes, stirring occasionally, until the onion is soft and light golden brown.

Tip the tomatoes into the pan, add the water and stir in the chilli, oregano and ketchup. Bring to a gentle simmer and cook for 15 minutes, stirring regularly. Serve it chunky like this or blitz with a stick blender for a smoother sauce – up to you. Keep the sauce warm until your meatloaf is ready.

Turn the meatloaf out on to a warmed plate or board and peel off the baking parchment. Cut it into thick slices and serve with the spicy sauce for pouring. Garnish with more parsley if you like.

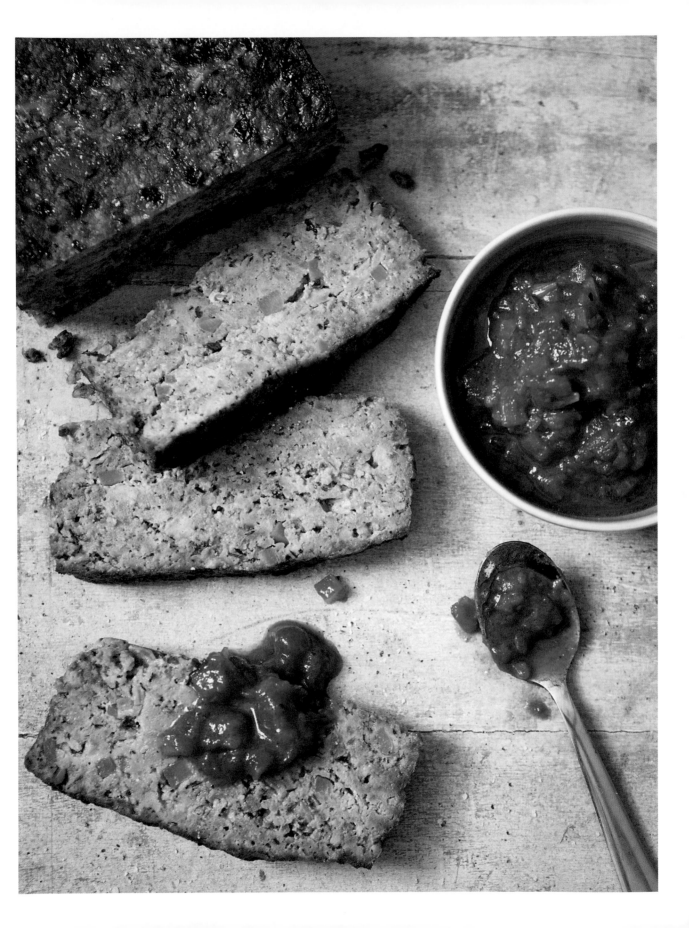

LOW-FAT BEEF RAVIOLI
WITH TOMATO SAUCE

337 calories per portion

These do take a bit of time to prepare but are well worth it and our special dough is lower in calories than the usual. You can make the filling and tomato sauce in advance, then mix the dough and make the ravioli later on. You could also serve the ravioli Italian style in a clear soup – in brodo.

Serves 6
Prep: 1 hour 15 minutes
Cooking time: 45–50 minutes

Special pasta dough
300g strong white flour, plus extra
    for rolling
½ tsp fine sea salt
200ml just-boiled water

Filling
1 small onion, chopped
2 garlic cloves, crushed
250g extra-lean minced beef
50ml red wine
300ml beef stock, made with
    ½ stock cube
2 tbsp tomato purée
1 tsp dried oregano
3 tbsp fine dried white breadcrumbs
flaked sea salt
freshly ground black pepper

Sauce
1 medium onion, finely chopped
2 garlic cloves, crushed
400g can of chopped tomatoes
100ml red wine
150ml water
1 tsp dried oregano
good pinch of dried chilli flakes
1 tsp caster sugar
2 tbsp half-fat crème fraiche
fresh basil leaves, to garnish
25g grated Parmesan, to serve

First make the special dough for the ravioli. Sift the flour and mix in the salt. Stir in the boiling water with a knife until a ball forms. If the dough seems too wet, add a bit more flour; if it's too dry, add more boiling water. Cover the dough and leave it to stand and cool for about an hour while you make the filling.

Put the onion, garlic and minced beef in a medium non-stick saucepan and dry-fry for 4–5 minutes. Keep stirring and squishing the meat against the sides of the pan to break up any clumps.

Stir in the wine, stock, tomato purée and oregano. Season with salt and pepper and bring everything to a gentle simmer. Cook for 20 minutes, stirring occasionally, until the beef and vegetables are tender. Tip it all out on to a plate, spread fairly thinly and leave to cool for 20 minutes.

While the filling is cooling, make the sauce. Put the onion, garlic, chopped tomatoes, wine, water, oregano, chilli and sugar in a medium non-stick pan and bring to a simmer. Cook over a low heat for 25–30 minutes or until the onion is tender and the liquid is well reduced, stirring occasionally. Blitz until smooth with a stick blender – or cool for a short while and blitz in a food processor. Press through a sieve into a clean saucepan to make a smooth purée. Stir in the crème fraiche and set aside.

Put the cooled filling in a food processor with the breadcrumbs and blitz to make a thick purée. You may need to remove the lid and push the mixture down a couple of times with a rubber spatula.

Place the rested dough on a lightly floured surface and knead for 5 minutes until it's very elastic. Take a third of the dough and divide it into 10 portions. Shape one portion into a ball and roll it out thinly on a floured surface into a rough circle of about 10cm, turning it as you go. The dough should be about 2mm thick. (Keep the rest of the portions of dough covered to prevent them from drying out.) Cut the circle into a neat disc with a 10cm fluted pastry cutter and set it aside. Repeat with the rest of the dough, keeping the cut circles lightly dusted with flour to stop them sticking to each other.

Take a disc of dough and lay it flat on the work surface. Place a heaped teaspoonful of the filling on one side of it. Dip your fingertip in a little cold water and rub around the edge. Fold the empty half over filling to form a semi-circle. Press the edges firmly together to seal, squeezing out any air as you go, then set it aside on a floured tray while you make the rest of the ravioli in the same way. You should end up with 30.

Half fill a very large saucepan with cold water, stir in a good pinch of salt and bring to the boil. Drop the ravioli gently into the hot water and bring it back to the boil. Cook for 8 minutes or until the pasta is tender, stirring occasionally. Warm the tomato sauce over a medium heat, stirring.

Drain the pasta in a colander and divide between warmed deep plates. Spoon over the hot tomato sauce, garnish with fresh basil and a sprinkling of Parmesan. Serve with a large, lightly dressed mixed salad on the side if you like.

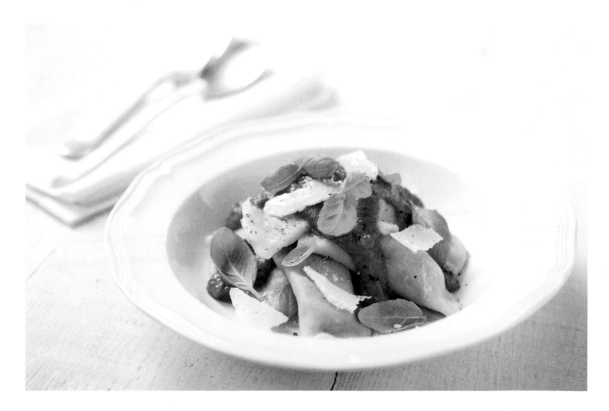

BEEF GOULASH

306 calories per portion

Lots of peppers and paprika make a good bit of braising steak into something special. A great foot-stomping feast from Hungary to stop you feeling hungry!

Serves 6
Prep: 20 minutes
Cooking time: 2 hours and
35 minutes

1kg good braising steak, preferably
   chuck steak
1 tbsp sunflower oil
3 medium onions, cut into
   12 wedges
3 garlic cloves, crushed
2 tsp hot smoked paprika
1 tbsp paprika
1 beef stock cube (Oxo works
   well here)
600ml cold water
400g can of chopped tomatoes
2 tbsp tomato purée
2 bay leaves
1 red pepper
1 green pepper
1 orange pepper
flaked sea salt
freshly ground black pepper

Preheat the oven to 170°C/Fan 150°C/Gas 3½. Trim any hard fat off the beef and cut the meat into rough 4cm chunks. Season well with salt and freshly ground black pepper.

Heat the oil in a large flameproof casserole dish. Add the steak and fry over a high heat until nicely browned all over, turning regularly. Tip the onions into the pan and cook with the beef for 5 minutes until softened. Add the crushed garlic and cook for a further minute, stirring regularly.

Sprinkle both paprikas over the meat and crumble the beef stock cube on top. Add the water, tomatoes, tomato purée and bay leaves. Season with salt and pepper, stir well and bring to a simmer. Cover with a tightly fitting lid and transfer the dish to the oven. Cook for 1½ hours.

While the beef is cooking, remove the core and seeds from each pepper and chuck them away. Cut each pepper into chunks of about 3cm. When the beef has cooked for 1½ hours, carefully remove the dish from the oven. Stir in the peppers, put the lid back on and put the goulash back in the oven for a further hour or until the beef is meltingly tender.

Serve with small portions of rice (see pages 178–179) and spoonfuls of soured cream if you like, but don't be too generous – soured cream contains less fat than double cream but still has 30 calories per tablespoon!

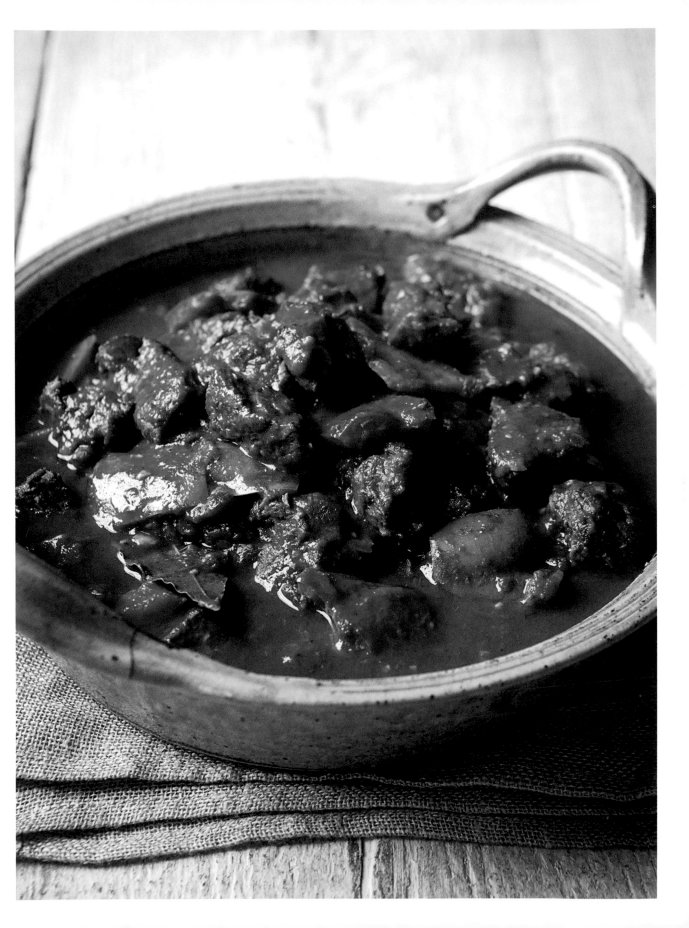

RICH BEEF IN RED WINE

416 calories per portion

Our take on a beef bourguignon – this tastes richer than Bill Gates. Perfect for a party, as you can do most of the preparation in advance.

Serves 6
Prep: 15 minutes
Cooking time: 2 hours and
22 minutes

1.25kg good braising steak,
    preferably chuck steak
150g rindless lean smoked back
    bacon (about 5 rashers)
1 tbsp sunflower oil
2 medium onions, finely chopped
3 garlic cloves, crushed
300ml red wine
2 tbsp tomato purée
500ml cold water
1 beef stock cube
2 large bay leaves
3 bushy sprigs of thyme
400g small shallots
250g button chestnut mushrooms,
    wiped and halved
2 tbsp cornflour
2 tbsp cold water
freshly chopped parsley, to garnish
    (optional)
flaked sea salt
freshly ground black pepper

Preheat the oven to 170°C/Fan 150°C/Gas 3½. Trim the braising steak of any hard fat and cut it into chunky pieces, each about 4cm. Season the beef really well with salt and freshly ground black pepper. Trim the bacon of any visible fat and cut it into 2cm-wide strips.

Heat the oil in a large flameproof casserole dish. Fry the beef and bacon over a medium-high heat for 3 minutes until lightly browned on all sides, turning every now and then.

Add the onion and garlic to the dish and fry for 2 minutes more. Pour over the wine and stir in the tomato purée and water. Crumble over the stock cube, add the herbs and bring to a simmer. Stir well, cover with a lid and transfer to the oven. Cook for 1½ hours.

While the beef is cooking, peel the shallots. Put the shallots in a heatproof bowl and cover with just-boiled water. Leave to stand for 5 minutes then drain. When the shallots are cool enough to handle, trim off the root close to the end so they don't fall apart and peel off the skin. Set aside.

Take the casserole dish out of the oven and stir in the shallots and mushrooms. Return to the oven for a further 45 minutes or until the beef is completely tender.

Mix the cornflour with the 2 tablespoons of water until smooth and stir this into the casserole. Place the dish on the hob and simmer for 1–2 minutes until thickened, stirring occasionally. Don't stir too much or the beef could fall apart.

Adjust the seasoning to taste, sprinkle with freshly chopped parsley and serve with small portions of rice or mashed potatoes and green beans. Colcannon (see page 181) goes well with this casserole too.

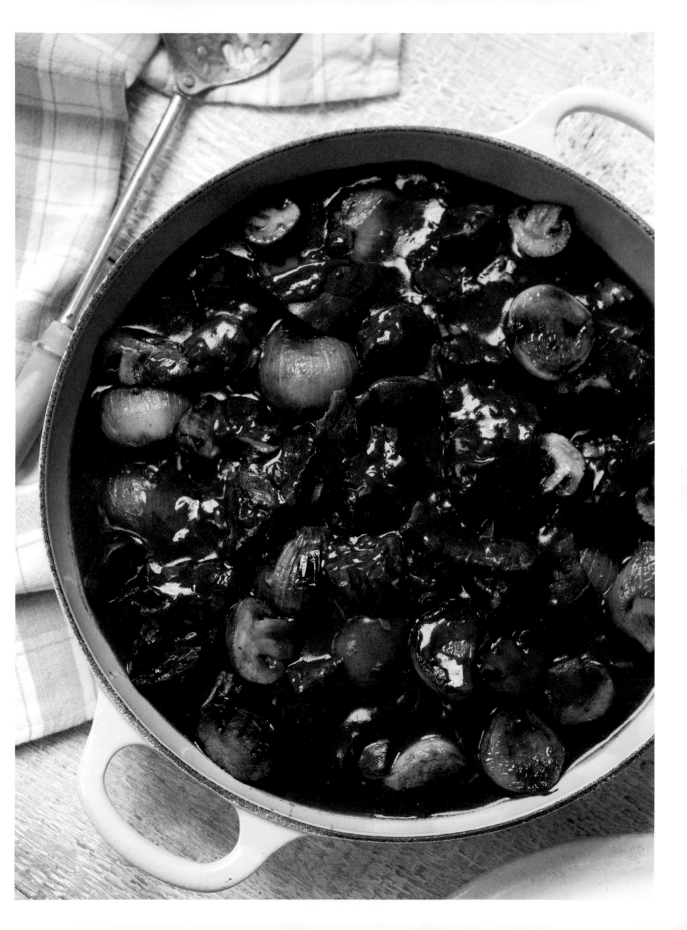

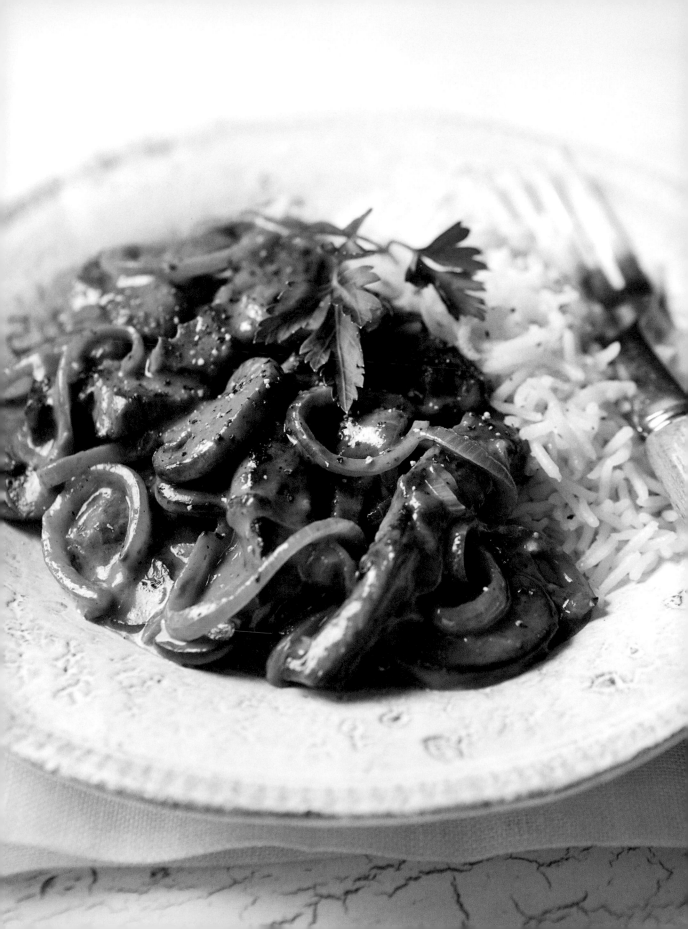

BEEF STROGANOFF

269 calories per portion (if serving 3); 202 calories per portion (if serving 4)

Our lower-calorie version of the classic, with half-fat crème fraiche and lots of mushrooms, makes a small amount of meat go a long way. And it tastes good.

Trim all the fat off the steak and slice it on a slight diagonal into long strips about 5mm thick. Season well with flaked sea salt and heaps of freshly ground black pepper.

Heat the oil in a large non-stick frying pan or wok and stir-fry the mushrooms and onions over a high heat for 5 minutes until softened and well browned. The colour will add lots of flavour but make sure they don't burn! Transfer the mushrooms and onions to a plate using a slotted spoon. Add the steak strips to the pan and stir-fry for 1–2 minutes until nicely browned but not cooked through. Transfer the meat to another plate.

Pour the 300ml of cold water into the pan and bring it to the boil. Crumble the stock cube into the boiling water and simmer for a minute, stirring. Mix the cornflour with 1 tablespoon of cold water until smooth and stir the mixture into the stock. Simmer for 30 seconds, stirring.

Put the mushrooms and onions back in the pan and continue to simmer for a minute until the sauce has thickened. Add the crème fraiche and when the sauce has combined, put the beef back in the pan and cook for a few seconds more until hot, while stirring.

Scatter with the fresh parsley and serve with small portions of freshly cooked rice (see pages 178–179).

Serves 3–4
Prep: 10 minutes
Cooking time: 10 minutes

1 large sirloin steak (about 350g)
1 tbsp sunflower oil
250g chestnut mushrooms, wiped and sliced
2 medium onions, halved and cut into thin wedges
300ml cold water, plus 1 tbsp
1 beef stock cube (Oxo is great for this dish)
2 tsp cornflour
3 tbsp half-fat crème fraiche
freshly chopped flatleaf parsley, to garnish
flaked sea salt
freshly ground black pepper

MORE FAB FAKEAWAYS

"We all live busy lives these days and takeaways have become a fact of life. Some nights you just can't get the thought of a kebab or a chicken curry out of your mind. Fear not! We have the solution to these moments of temptation: more of our fab fakeaways. Enjoy chicken tikka masala, beef Madras – and wait until you taste our version of a doner kebab! Don't let the takeaway take over your diet, but you can enjoy a fakeaway any night of the week. "

——— Dave ———

CREAMY PRAWN KORMA

273 calories per portion (if serving 3); 205 calories per portion (if serving 4)

Ready in no time, this korma will satisfy your takeaway yearnings. Rich, creamy and satisfying – absolutely prawnographic.

Serves 3–4
Prep: 10 minutes
Cooking time: 20–25 minutes

1 tbsp sunflower oil
2 medium onions, finely chopped
4 garlic cloves, finely sliced
20g chunk of fresh root ginger, peeled and finely chopped
3 tbsp Korma curry paste
500ml cold water
2 tbsp double or single cream
2 tsp caster sugar
400g peeled raw tiger prawns, deveined if necessary and thawed if frozen
20g bunch of fresh coriander, leaves roughly chopped
flaked sea salt

Heat the oil in a medium non-stick saucepan or sauté pan and stir in the onions, garlic and ginger. Cover the pan with a lid and cook the onions and garlic over a medium heat for 10 minutes until pale golden brown, stirring occasionally.

Remove the lid and stir in the curry paste. Cook for a further minute, while stirring, then add the water and bring to the boil. Lower the heat slightly and simmer for 8–10 minutes, uncovered, until the liquid has reduced by half and the onions are very soft.

Remove the pan from the heat and, using a stick blender, blitz to a smooth sauce. Stir in the cream and sugar, season with a little salt and put the pan back on the heat.

Add the prawns to the pan, bring to a simmer and cook for 3–4 minutes, stirring, until the prawns are completely pink and beginning to curl.

Sprinkle the fresh coriander over the top, stir well and serve the korma immediately with a small portion of rice.

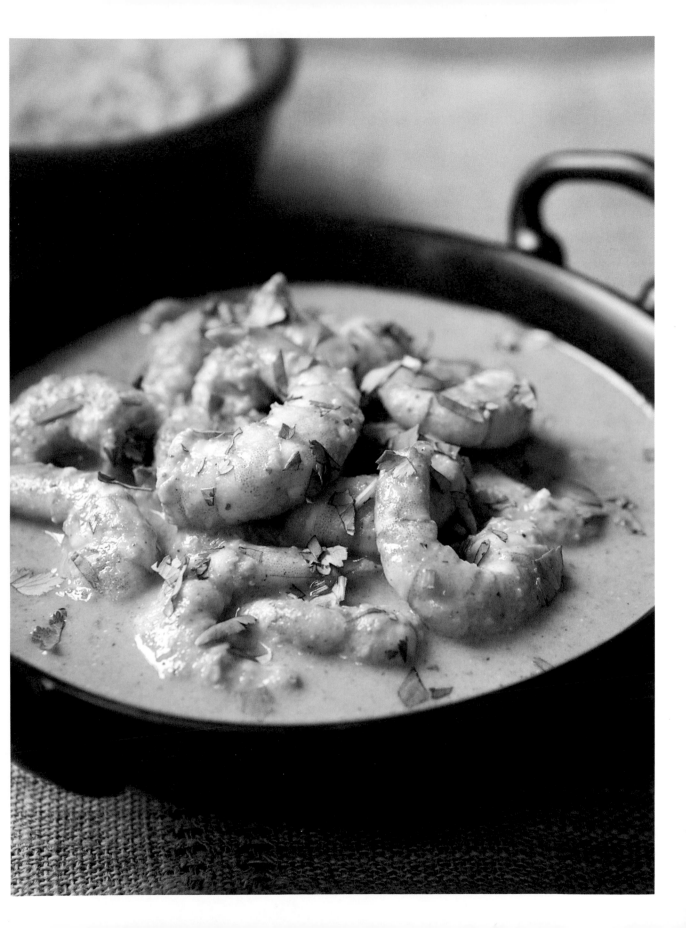

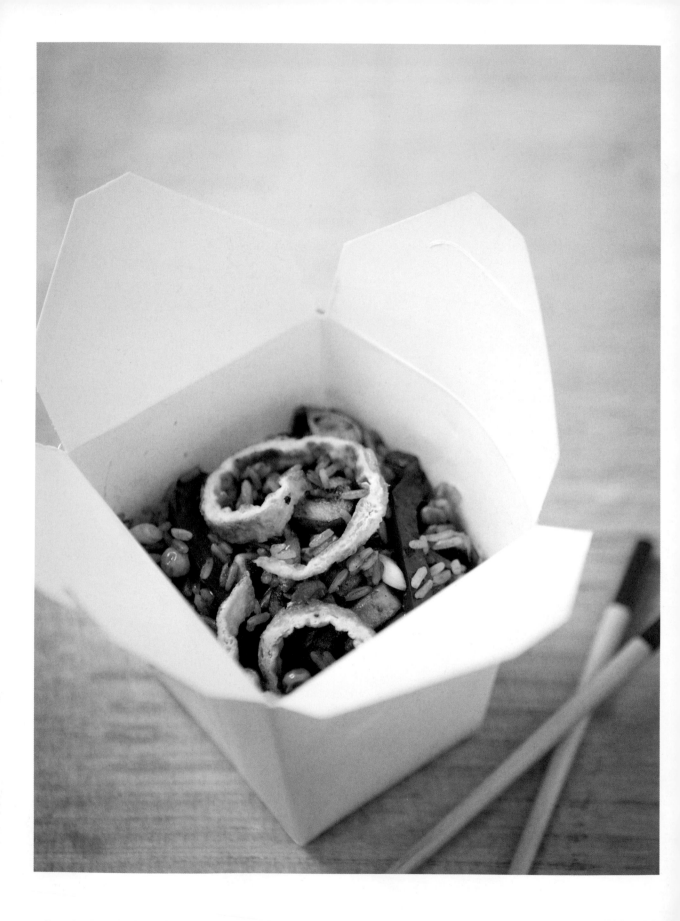

EGG FRIED RICE

304 calories per portion

A quick and easy supper dish. Add a few prawns or even some cooked, sliced chicken or pork left over from a roast if you like, but don't forget to take the extra calories into account. If you don't fancy making the omelette, just stir the beaten eggs into the stir-fried vegetables and cook for a few seconds before adding the hot rice and soy sauce.

Half fill a medium saucepan with water and bring it to the boil. Add the rice, bring the water back to the boil, then cook for 10–12 minutes or until the rice is tender, stirring occasionally.

While the rice is cooking, mist a large non-stick frying pan with oil and put it on a medium-high heat. Season the beaten eggs with some salt and pepper. Pour the eggs into the pan and swirl them around so they cover the base to make a thin omelette. Cook for 2 minutes, then turn the omelette over with a heatproof palette knife and cook on the other side for a further minute. Slide the omelette on to a plate, cut it into 1cm-wide strips and set aside. Drain the rice in a large sieve.

Put the frying pan back on the heat and mist with more oil. Stir-fry the pepper and mushrooms for 3 minutes until softened and lightly browned, then add the peas and cook for another minute, stirring. Add the spring onions, garlic and ginger to the pan and cook for a minute more, stirring constantly and spraying with a little more oil if necessary.

Tip the rice and sliced omelette into the frying pan, pour over the soy sauce and toss with the vegetables until everything is well mixed together. Heat through for a minute or so until the omelette is hot, then serve.

Serves 2
Prep: 10 minutes
Cooking time: 16–18 minutes

75g easy-cook long-grain rice, such as Uncle Ben's

oil, for spraying

2 medium eggs, beaten

1 red pepper, deseeded and thinly sliced

100g small chestnut mushrooms, wiped and sliced

50g frozen peas

6 spring onions, trimmed and sliced

2 garlic cloves, crushed

20g chunk of fresh root ginger, peeled and finely grated

2 tbsp dark soy sauce

flaked sea salt

freshly ground black pepper

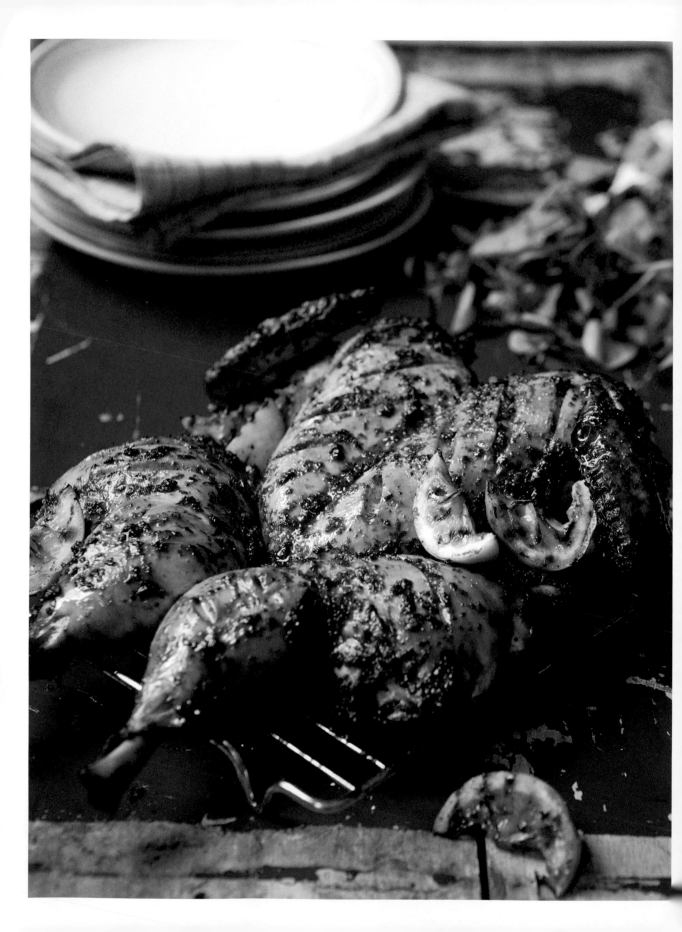

PIRI PIRI CHICKEN

369 calories per portion (if serving 4); 295 calories per portion (if serving 5)

Piri piri is all the rage at the moment. This delicious, moist chicken has a spicy marinade and you can add more bird's-eye chillies if you like your food hot, hot, hot. If you don't fancy preparing the whole chicken, use skinless chicken thighs and breasts instead and bake them for 20–30 minutes.

To make the marinade, put all the ingredients in a food processor and blitz until everything is well mixed and chopped up small. Now you need to spatchcock the chicken by removing the backbone but leaving it whole. Turn the bird on to its breast and carefully cut either side of the backbone with good scissors or poultry shears. Discard the bone. Cut off the foot joints and wing tips.

Strip off all the skin from the bird apart from the ends of the wings, which are easier to remove after cooking. You'll find it simpler to do this if you snip the membrane between the skin and the chicken flesh as you go. Snip off any obvious fat with scissors – it will be a creamy white colour.

Open the chicken out and place it on the board so the breast side is facing upwards. Press down heavily with the palms of your hands to break the breastbone and flatten the chicken as evenly as possible. This will help it cook more quickly. Don't worry if you can't press hard enough to break the breastbone – as long as the chicken looks flat, it will cook evenly. Using a sharp knife, slash through the thickest parts of the legs and breasts. Place the chicken in a shallow non-metallic dish – a lasagne dish is ideal – and tuck in the legs and wings.

Spoon over all the marinade and really massage it into both sides of the chicken, ensuring that every bit of it is well coated. Cover the dish with cling film and leave the chicken to marinate in the fridge for at least 4 hours or ideally overnight.

Preheat the oven to 210°C/Fan 190°C/Gas 6½. Take the chicken out of the dish and place it on a rack inside a large baking tray, breast-side up. Roast for 50–60 minutes until lightly browned and cooked through. The juices should run clear when the thickest part of a thigh is pierced with a skewer. Cover the chicken loosely with foil and leave it to rest for 10 minutes before carving. Add a garnish of watercress and some lemon wedges for squeezing.

Serves 4–5
Prep: 20 minutes, plus marinating
Cooking time: 50–60 minutes

1 large fresh chicken, about 2kg
fresh watercress, to garnish
lemon wedges, to serve

Piri piri marinade
4 plump red chillies, deseeded and
   roughly chopped
2 red bird's-eye chillies, stalks
   removed, sliced
4 garlic cloves, peeled and halved
20g bunch of flatleaf parsley
   (with stalks)
juice of 2 lemons, about 65ml
2 tbsp white wine vinegar
1 tsp smoked paprika, sweet or hot
1 tsp oregano
1 tsp caster sugar
2 tsp flaked sea salt

JERK CHICKEN

333 calories per portion (if serving 4); 222 calories per portion (if serving 6)

We've always loved hot spicy food but we've loved it even more since starting to watch our weight. Spice and chilli add flavour without flab. If you can't get hold of scotch bonnet chillies, use two red bird's-eye chillies and two plump or long red chillies instead. But don't deseed them – you need the heat for this marinade. Jamaiking me hungry already!

Serves 4–6
Prep: 15 minutes, plus marinating
Cooking time: 25 minutes

12 boneless, skinless chicken thighs
lime wedges, to serve
flaked sea salt
freshly ground black pepper

Marinade
6 spring onions, trimmed and
    roughly chopped
20g chunk of fresh root ginger,
    peeled and roughly chopped
4 garlic cloves, peeled and halved
2–3 scotch bonnet chillies,
    stalks removed
1 tbsp fresh thyme leaves
    (or 1 tsp dried thyme)
1 tsp ground allspice
½ tsp ground nutmeg
½ tsp ground cinnamon
3 tbsp dark brown sugar
2 tbsp fresh lime juice
1½ tbsp dark soy sauce

To make the marinade, put all the ingredients in a food processor and blitz to make a thick purée. You'll need to remove the lid and push the mixture down a couple of times with a rubber spatula until you get the right consistency.

Put the chicken on a board and trim off as much fat as you can with good kitchen scissors. Slash each thigh a couple of times with a sharp knife, put them all in a bowl and season with a little salt and lots of freshly ground black pepper. Tip the jerk marinade on top and mix well, then cover and chill for at least 2 hours or overnight.

Preheat the oven to 220°C/Fan 200°C/Gas 7 and line a large baking tray with baking parchment. Place the chicken on the tray, shaking off any excess marinade as you go and shaping the pieces back into neat thighs if they have opened out during marinating.

Bake the chicken for 25 minutes or until it is all thoroughly cooked, deep golden brown and charred in places. Serve hot or cold with lime wedges for squeezing and a large mixed salad. You could also serve small portions of rice if you like (see pages 178–179).

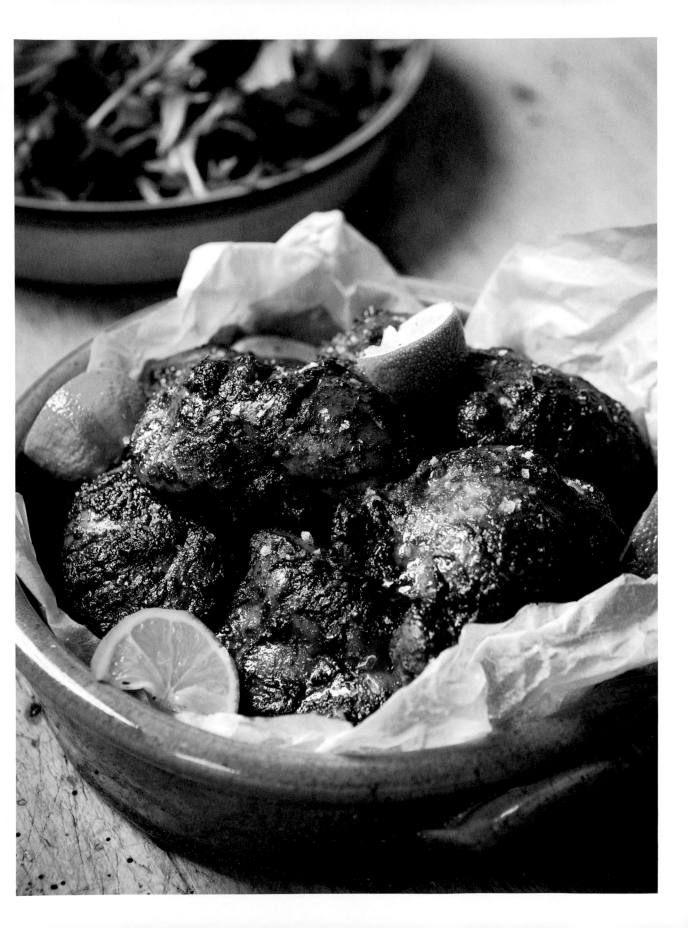

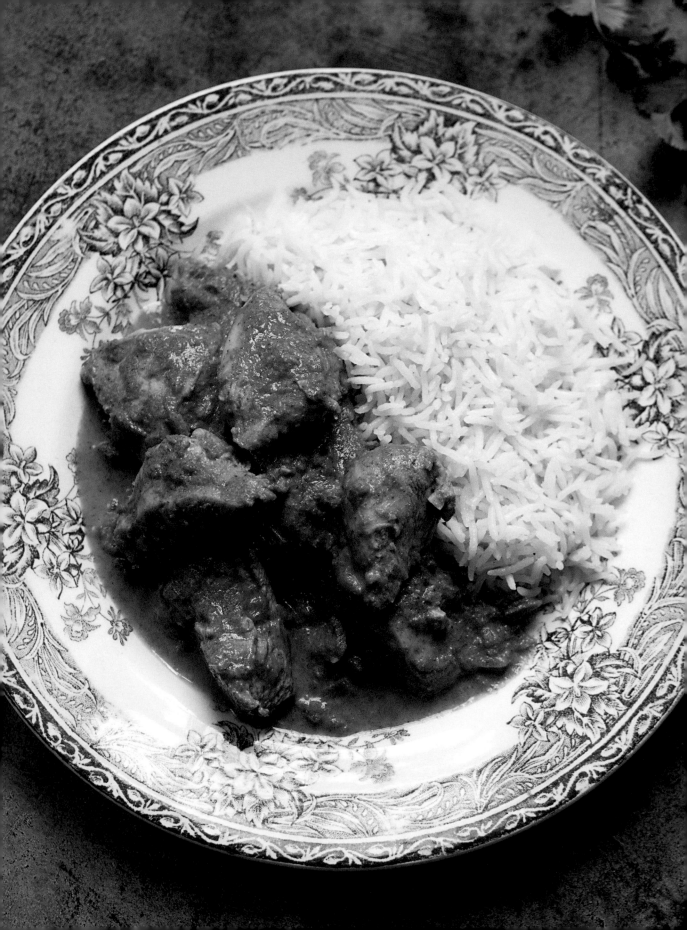

LOW-CAL CHICKEN TIKKA MASALA

302 calories per serving

Britain's favourite curry, chicken tikka masala can be a real diet buster but don't worry, you can relax and enjoy our version without guilt. Cuts calories but not flavour.

To make the marinade, mix the curry powder, paprika and salt in a large bowl. Add the ginger, garlic and yoghurt and stir until well combined. Cut each chicken breast into 7–9 pieces. Stir the chicken pieces into the marinade and mix until the chicken is well coated. Cover, chill and leave to marinate for at least 1 hour but ideally up to 4 hours or even overnight.

While the chicken is marinating, make the sauce. Heat the oil in a large non-stick saucepan. Tip the onions, garlic and ginger into the pan, cover with a lid and gently fry for 10 minutes, until the onions are lightly browned and very soft, stirring occasionally.

Add the curry powder to the pan and cook for 2 minutes, stirring frequently. Add the tomato purée, caster sugar and salt and fry for a further 30 seconds, stirring constantly.

Pour the 350ml of water into the pan, and simmer gently for 5 minutes, stirring occasionally. Remove the pan from the heat and use a hand blender to blitz the sauce until as smooth as possible. Set aside.

Heat the teaspoon of oil in a large non-stick frying pan and stir-fry the marinated chicken for about 3 minutes over a medium-high heat until lightly coloured.

Pour your masala sauce into the pan, add the cream and cook for 3–4 minutes longer, stirring until the chicken is tender and cooked through, with no pinkness remaining. Add a little extra water if the sauce seems too thick.

Serve with some rice (see pages 178–179) and a large mixed salad if you like and garnish with some fresh coriander sprigs.

Serves 4
Prep: 30 minutes, plus marinating
Cooking time: about 25 minutes

---

4 boneless, skinless chicken breasts (about 150g each)
1 tsp sunflower oil

Marinade
2 tbsp medium curry powder
1½ tsp smoked paprika (not hot smoked)
1 tsp flaked sea salt
15g chunk of fresh root ginger, peeled and finely grated
2 garlic cloves, crushed
6 tbsp plain fat-free yoghurt

Sauce
1 tbsp sunflower oil
2 medium onions, chopped
2 garlic cloves, crushed
15g chunk of fresh root ginger, peeled and finely grated
1 tbsp medium curry powder
2 tbsp tomato purée
2 tsp caster sugar
1 tsp flaked sea salt
350ml cold water
2 tbsp double or single cream
fresh coriander sprigs, to garnish

CHICKEN BHUNA

305 calories per portion

A great addition to your light curry repertoire, this makes the perfect answer to takeaway cravings. Leave the chilli powder out if you prefer a mild curry, and serve with a small portion of freshly cooked long-grain or basmati rice if you like. Allow about 50 grams of dry rice per person – and bear in mind that you'll add about another 180 calories per serving.

Serves 4
Prep: 15 minutes
Cooking time: 40 minutes

8 boneless, skinless chicken thighs
1 x red, orange and green pepper
40g chunk of fresh root ginger, peeled
2 medium onions, quartered
4 garlic cloves, peeled
2 tsp mild curry powder
2 tsp garam masala
½ tsp hot chilli powder (optional)
1 tbsp sunflower oil
400g can of chopped tomatoes
600ml chicken stock, made with 1 stock cube
1 tbsp caster sugar
1 tbsp cornflour
2 tbsp cold water
fresh coriander, to garnish (optional)
flaked sea salt
freshly ground black pepper

Put the chicken thighs on a board and trim off any visible fat with good kitchen scissors, then cut each chicken thigh into 3 pieces. Season with lots of freshly ground black pepper. Deseed the peppers and cut them into chunks of about 3cm. Set aside.

Cut the ginger into small pieces and put them in a food processor. Add the onion quarters, garlic, curry powder, garam masala and chilli powder, then blitz until everything is as finely blended as possible. You may need to remove the lid and push the mixture down with a rubber spatula once or twice until it reaches the right consistency. If you don't have a food processor, coarsely grate the onion and finely grate the ginger and garlic, then mix with the spices in a bowl.

Heat the oil in a large non-stick saucepan. Add the spiced onion paste and cook it over a medium heat for 10 minutes until softened and lightly browned, stirring regularly. Tip the tomatoes into the pan and cook for 5 minutes, stirring constantly.

Add the chicken and peppers to the curry sauce and cook for 2 minutes, stirring. Add the chicken stock and sugar. Bring to a gentle simmer and cook for 20 minutes or until the chicken is tender, stirring occasionally.

Mix the cornflour with the water and stir the mixture into the sauce. Simmer for another 2–3 minutes until the sauce has thickened, stirring occasionally. Season with salt and pepper to taste and serve garnished with fresh coriander if you like.

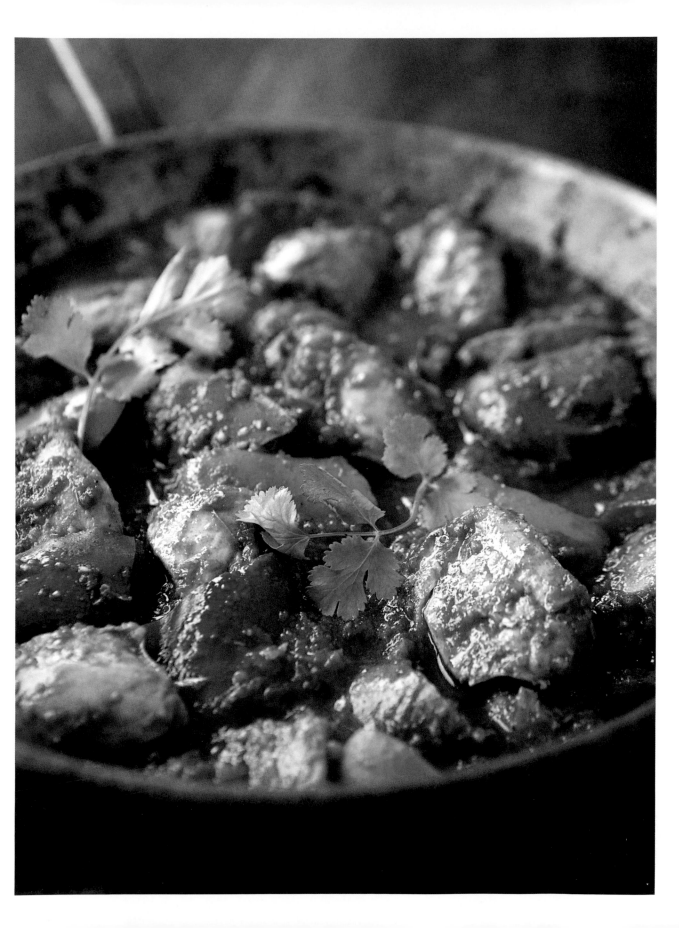

CHICKEN BIRYANI

380 calories per portion (if serving 5); 317 calories per portion (if serving 6)

Another of our favourites. We've upped the veg content on this and cut down on the rice so we can still include biryani on our menu. You're going to love it just as much as we do.

Serves 5–6
Prep: 20 minutes
Cooking time: 50 minutes

100ml semi-skimmed milk
pinch of saffron strands
200g basmati rice
8 boneless, skinless chicken thighs
1 tbsp sunflower oil
2 medium onions, finely sliced
2 red peppers, deseeded and cut
  into 2.5cm chunks
4 garlic cloves, finely sliced
25g chunk of fresh root ginger,
  peeled and finely chopped
1 plump fresh red chilli, finely
  chopped (or 1 tsp dried
  chilli flakes)
1 tbsp garam masala
6 cloves
10 cardamom pods, lightly crushed
80–100g bag of young
  spinach leaves
400ml chicken stock, made
  with 1 stock cube
flaked sea salt
freshly ground black pepper

Pour the milk into a small saucepan, add the saffron strands and heat gently for 2–3 minutes without boiling. Remove from the heat and set aside.

Preheat the oven to 190°C/Fan 170°C/Gas 5. Half fill a large pan with water and bring it to the boil. Put the rice in a sieve and rinse under plenty of cold water, then stir it into the hot water and bring it back to the boil. Cook for 5 minutes, then drain well in the sieve and set aside.

Remove any visible fat from the chicken thighs and cut each thigh into 4 pieces. Season well with salt and ground black pepper. Heat the oil in a large, wide based non-stick saucepan or sauté pan.

Fry the chicken over a medium-high heat for 3 minutes, turning it regularly. Transfer the chicken to a plate using a slotted spoon and put the pan back on the heat. Add the onion and fry for 5 minutes until lightly browned and beginning to crisp, stirring often. Reduce the heat slightly, add the peppers, garlic, ginger and chilli and cook for 2 minutes more, while stirring. Sprinkle over the garam masala, cloves and cardamom and cook for 1 minute, continuing to stir.

Tip the chicken back into the pan and toss with the vegetables and spices. Stir in the baby spinach, stock and rice and remove from the heat. Stir in the saffron milk.

Carefully transfer the chicken, vegetables and rice into a large ovenproof dish that will hold at least 2 litres. A lasagne dish is perfect, but a roasting tin will do. Heap it up a little in the middle.

Cover the dish with a layer of tightly fitting foil. Bake for 30 minutes or until the rice is tender and all the liquid has been absorbed. Remove the foil, fluff up the rice with a fork and take to the table! Warn everyone not to eat the cloves or cardamom pods!

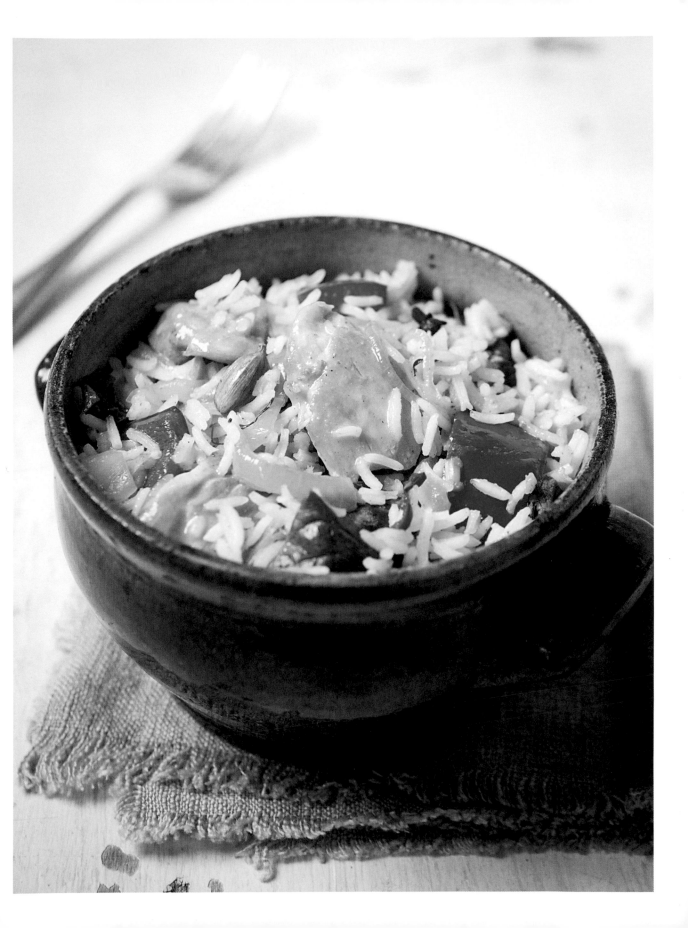

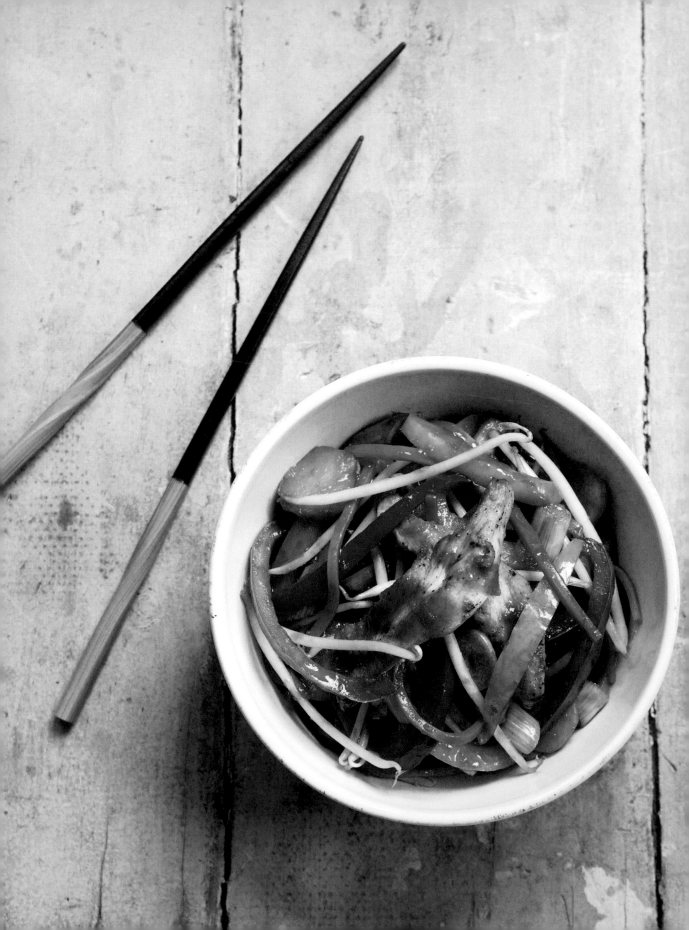

CHICKEN CHOW MEIN

292 calories per portion

Use enough beansprouts in our dieter's version of chow mein and we bet no one will notice there aren't any noodles! Make sure you slice the chicken really thinly so it cooks quickly and check that it is cooked through, and no pinkness remains, before serving.

Mix the sugar and cornflour together and slowly stir in the soy sauce, sherry and water. Put to one side while you prepare all your vegetables.

Heat the oil in a large non-stick frying pan or wok. Stir-fry the thinly sliced chicken over a high heat for 2–3 minutes until it is beginning to brown slightly. Add the peppers and carrots and stir-fry for 2 minutes.

Scatter the ginger, garlic, spring onions and water chestnuts into the pan. Season with lots of freshly ground black pepper and stir-fry together for 2 minutes.

Stir the soy mixture to mix the ingredients again, then pour it into the pan. Add the beansprouts and toss everything together for 1–2 minutes until hot and glossy. Check that the chicken is cooked through, then serve at once.

Serves 4
Prep: 20 minutes
Cooking time: 9 minutes

1 tbsp soft light brown sugar
2 tsp cornflour
2 tbsp dark soy sauce
2 tbsp dry sherry
100ml water
2 tbsp sunflower oil
3 boneless, skinless chicken breasts (each about 150g), thinly sliced
1 red, 1 yellow and 1 green pepper, quartered, deseeded and sliced
2 medium carrots, peeled and thinly sliced
25g chunk of fresh root ginger, peeled and finely grated
3 garlic cloves, very finely sliced
10 spring onions, trimmed and cut into 1cm slices
225g can of water chestnuts, drained and halved
300g bag of beansprouts, rinsed and drained
freshly ground black pepper

DIETER'S DONER KEBABS

361 calories per portion

They said it couldn't be done but here it is – our version of everyone's favourite post-pub food. These kebabs taste just like the real thing, but have fewer than half the calories! Make sure you fill your pitta with lots of salady bits for extra colour and crunch and don't forget the chilli soss!

Serves 4
Prep: 20 minutes
Cooking time: 5 minutes

200g lean lamb leg steaks (probably 2 steaks)
200g lean minced lamb
½ medium onion, roughly chopped
1 tsp ground coriander
1 tsp ground cumin
1 tsp flaked sea salt
1 tsp plain flour
4 white or wholemeal pitta breads (each about 60g)
oil, for spraying
hot chilli sauce (optional)
freshly ground black pepper

Garlic sauce
4 tbsp fat-free yoghurt
1 large garlic clove, crushed
pinch of flaked sea salt

Salad
2 large tomatoes, sliced
100g cucumber, sliced
shredded lettuce,
pickled chillies, finely shredded (optional)
white cabbage and red onion rings (optional)

To make the garlic sauce, mix all the ingredients in a small bowl and set aside to allow the flavours to mingle.

Trim the lamb steaks, removing any visible fat, and cut them into 3cm chunks. Put the lamb mince and steaks in a food processor with the onion, coriander, cumin, salt and lots of freshly ground black pepper. Blitz until as smooth as possible. You may need to remove the lid and push the mixture down a couple of times with a rubber spatula until it's the right consistency.

Divide the mince mixture into 4 balls. Cut a 60cm sheet of cling film and dust with ¼ teaspoon of sifted flour. Place a lamb portion on half of the film and fold the rest of the cling film over to cover it completely. Use a rolling pin to roll the kebab mixture thinly. Rolling this way will help stop the lamb sticking, but it will be delicate so take care not too roll it too thinly – about 5mm is just about right. Leave it inside the cling film. Do the same with the remaining portions of lamb.

Put the pitta breads on a baking tray and place them under a preheated medium grill – not too close – for 1–2 minutes on each side until hot. Keep warm. Mist a large non-stick frying pan with oil and place over a medium-high heat.

Lift the cling film off the top of a portion of lamb. Peel off the backing film and, holding the lamb on a spatula or over your hand, very gently and carefully place it in the hot frying pan. Do the same with a second piece of flattened lamb and fry both for about 1 minute on each side until lightly browned and cooked through. Flatten the lamb into the hot pan by pressing it with a spatula as the meat cooks. Put the lamb on a warmed plate and cook the other 2 portions.

Put the warmed pittas on a board and cut them open along one side, then fill with salad and the hot lamb. Spoon over the garlic sauce and chilli sauce too, if you like. Add a couple of pickled chillies for extra authenticity and serve!

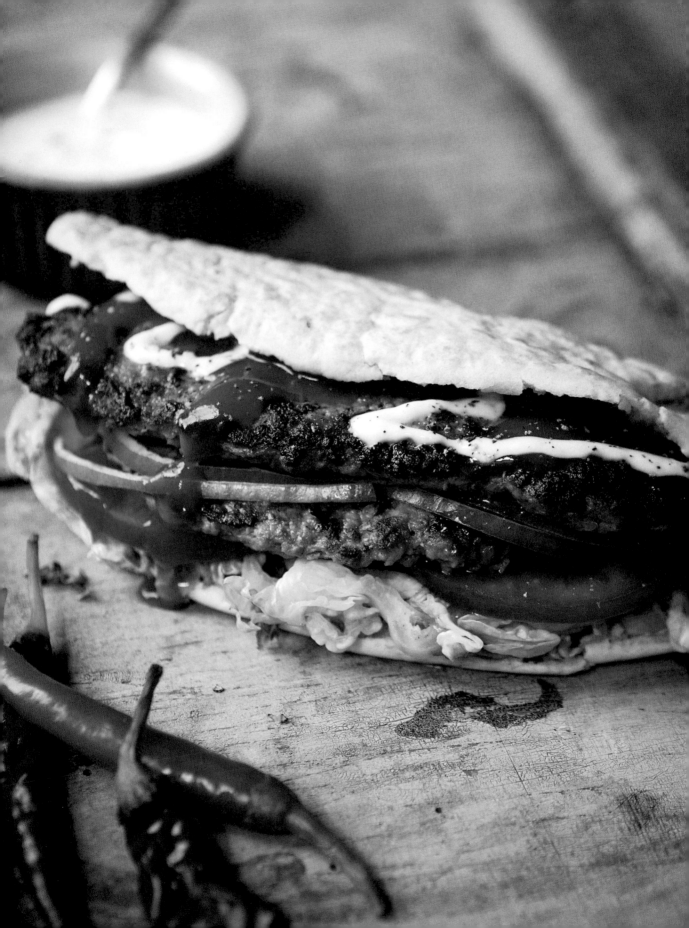

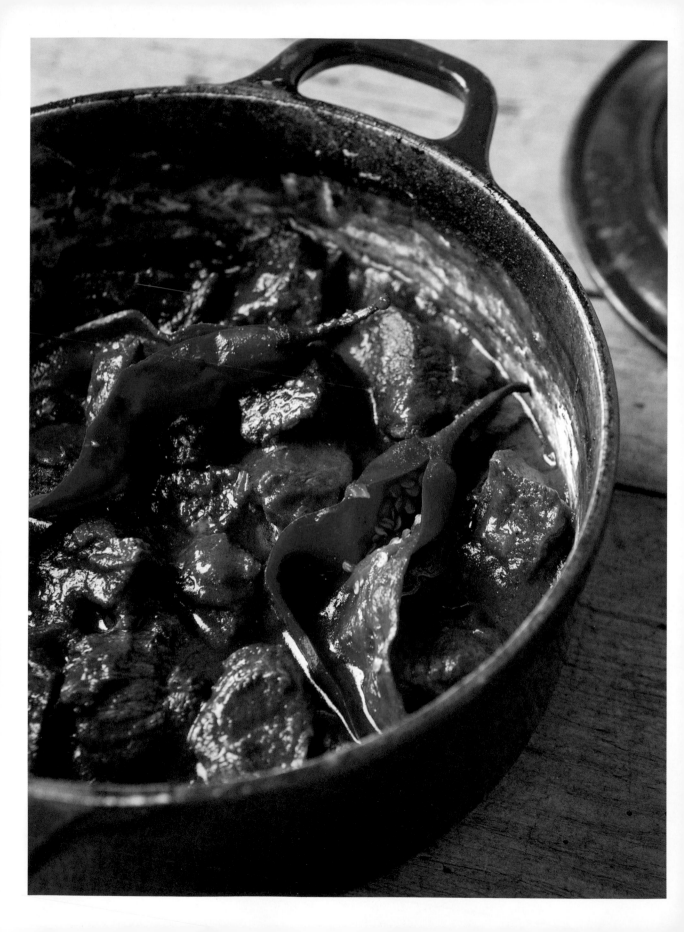

FIERY BEEF MADRAS

346 calories per portion

This is a rich, hot beef curry that's very easy to put together and will go down well with anyone who likes a bit of spice – like us. If you don't fancy beef, you can make the curry with 12 boneless, skinless chicken thighs and use chicken stock instead of beef.

Preheat the oven to 170°C/Fan 150°C/Gas 3½. Place the chillies on a board and finely chop 2 of them. Split the other 2 chillies from stalk to tip on one side without opening or removing the seeds. Remove any visible fat from the beef and cut the meat into chunks of about 3cm if it's not already cut.

Heat a large flameproof casserole dish on the hob. Add the oil and fry the onion, garlic and chopped chillies over a high heat for 1 minute, while stirring. Sprinkle over the curry powder and stir for a few seconds before adding the chopped tomatoes and tomato purée.

Cook over a medium-high heat for 5 minutes, stirring constantly until the liquid evaporates and the sauce looks very thick and deep red. Don't let the garlic or spices burn or they'll make the sauce taste bitter.

Next, add the beef, whole chillies, sugar and salt to the casserole dish and cook for 2 minutes, turning the beef regularly until lightly coloured and well coated in the tomato mixture.

Pour over the stock and bring to a simmer, stirring. Cover the dish with a lid and carefully transfer it to the oven. Cook for 1½–1¾ hours or until the beef is beautifully tender and the sauce has thickened. (If the sauce is still a little thin, put the casserole dish back on the hob and simmer for 2–3 minutes, stirring regularly.)

Serve with natural yoghurt and add a small portion of rice (see pages 178–179), or a couple of chapatis if you like, but remember to add on those extra calories.

Serves 4
Prep: 10 minutes
Cooking time: about 1 hour and 55 minutes

4 long red chillies
800g good braising steak
1 tbsp sunflower oil
½ medium onion, finely chopped
2 garlic cloves, crushed
2 tsp medium curry powder
400g can of chopped tomatoes
1 tbsp tomato purée
1 tsp caster sugar
1 tsp flaked sea salt
750ml beef stock, made
    with 1 stock cube
4 tbsp fat-free natural yoghurt,
    to serve

FOOD
FROM AFAR

"We Brits love a bit of exotic and we're passionate fans of dishes like satays, tagines and Thai salads. Dave and I have been lucky enough to do lots of travelling in our restless quest for amazing food to bring to you and we've been inspired by the cuisines of Asia, north Africa, the Caribbean and elsewhere. We've learned a lot about flavour from these styles of cookery and that's been a great help in developing our dieters' dishes. After all, there are no calories in taste, and food is all about taste. Turn your evening meal into a foreign holiday with our food from afar recipes – full-blown flavour but low in calories."

Si

LIGHT CHICKEN SATAY

283 calories per portion; 94 calories per skewer

Quick to make and as good as the real thing to eat, but don't forget to allow plenty of time for marinating. You can make beef or prawn versions too. Serve with a large salad.

Makes 10–12 skewers (serves 4)
Prep: 30 minutes, plus marinating
Cooking time: 4 minutes

3 boneless, skinless chicken breasts
    (each about 225g)

Marinade
2 lemon grass stalks, trimmed and
    white part roughly chopped
20g chunk of fresh root ginger,
    peeled and roughly chopped
3 garlic cloves, peeled
2 red bird's-eye chillies,
    stalks trimmed
2 tsp ground cumin
2 tsp ground coriander
½ tsp ground turmeric
1 tbsp light soft brown sugar
2 tsp dark soy sauce
2 tsp nam pla (Thai fish sauce)
1 tbsp fresh lime juice
1 tbsp sunflower oil, plus
    1 tsp for greasing
lime wedges, for squeezing
freshly ground black pepper

Peanut sauce
2 tbsp crunchy peanut butter
3 tbsp just-boiled water
1 tbsp Thai sweet chilli
    dipping sauce

First make the marinade. Put the lemon grass, ginger, garlic, chillies, spices, sugar, soy sauce, nam pla, lime juice and 1 tablespoon of oil in a food processor and blitz to make a paste. You may need to remove the lid a couple of times and push the mixture down with a rubber spatula until it's the right consistency. Scrape it all into a bowl and season with plenty of black pepper.

Trim any visible fat off the chicken breasts and cut them at a slight diagonal angle into 6 or 7 strips of about 8cm long. Add the strips to the marinade and stir well. Drain the skewers. Thread chicken strips on to each skewer, making sure not to thread them too tightly as the heat needs to penetrate. The chicken should be fairly flat so it cooks evenly once threaded. Put the skewers on a plate, cover and leave to marinate in the fridge for at least an hour or overnight.

To make the sauce, put the peanut butter in a small heatproof bowl and stir in the just-boiled water until evenly mixed. Add the sweet chilli sauce and stir well. Set aside.

Heat a large non-stick frying pan or griddle until it's very hot and brush with a little oil. Cook the satay for about 2 minutes on each side or until lightly browned and cooked throughout. Press the chicken down lightly with a spatula to ensure it has full contact with the hot surface.

If you prefer to grill the satay, place the skewers on a rack above a baking tray or a grill pan lined with foil. Cook under a preheated hot grill for the same time as above, turning once until lightly charred and cooked throughout. Serve the hot satay with the warm peanut sauce for dipping and lime wedges for a squeeze of tangy juice.

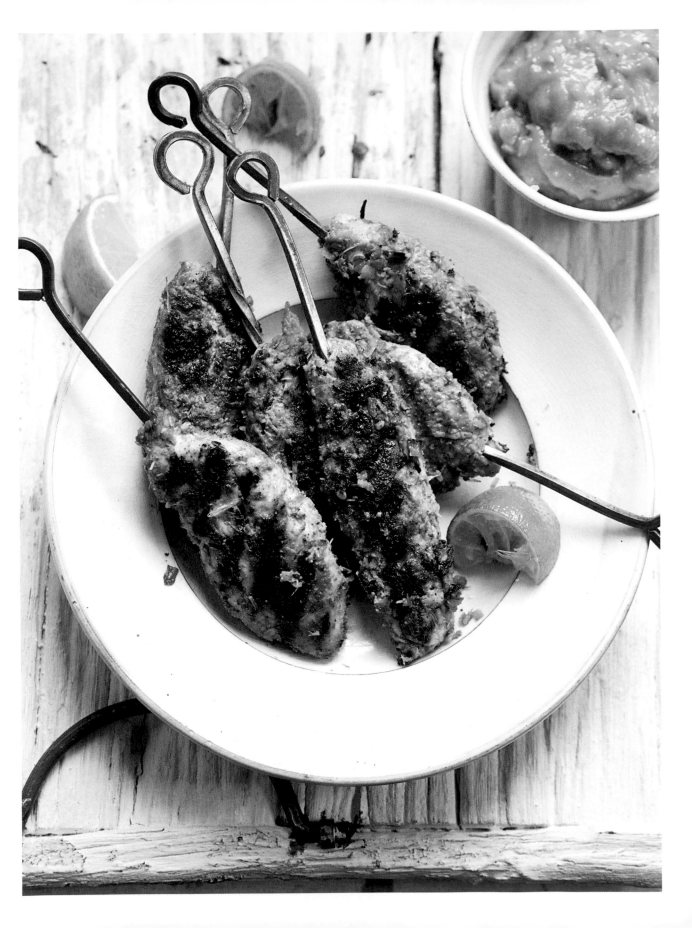

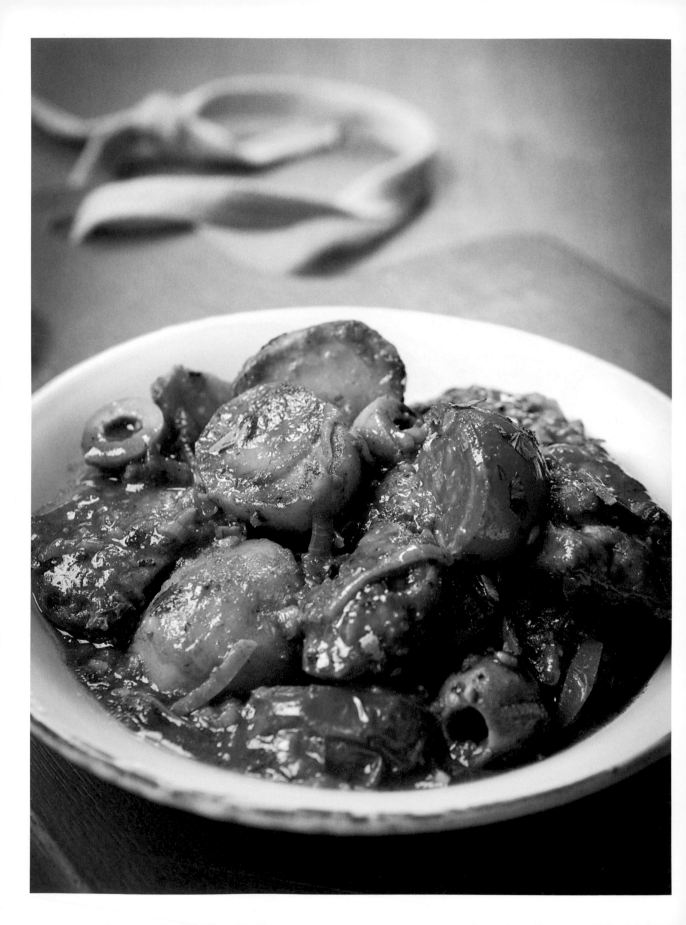

CHICKEN TAGINE WITH PRESERVED LEMONS

391 calories per portion (if serving 4); 313 calories per portion (if serving 5)

Saffron, chilli, preserved lemons, coriander – our version of this North African stew is a winner. It's fragrant, filling and fabulous, so enjoy. You can buy jars of preserved lemons in large supermarkets.

Put the saffron in a measuring jug with the stock cube and pour over the 250ml of just-boiled water. Stir until the stock cube dissolves and set aside. Put the chicken thighs on a board and trim off all the visible fat, then season the chicken with salt and pepper. Slice the preserved lemons into very thin strips, flicking out any pips as you go.

Heat the oil in a large non-stick saucepan. Add the onions, garlic, ginger, cumin, paprika and chilli flakes. Season with lots of black pepper and cook for 2 minutes, while stirring. Add the 2 tablespoons of cold water and steam-fry for another 3 minutes, stirring regularly until the onions are lightly browned. Add the chicken and preserved lemons to the saucepan and cook over a medium heat for 5 minutes, turning the chicken until it's lightly coloured on all sides.

Meanwhile, peel the potatoes and cut them into rough wedge shapes or chunks of about 4cm. Roughly chop the tomatoes and cut the pitted olives in half. Put the potatoes, tomatoes and olives in a large bowl and toss with the herbs and plenty of salt and pepper.

Scatter the vegetable mix over the chicken, pour over the saffron stock and cover the pan tightly with a lid. Simmer over a very low heat for 35–40 minutes, without removing the lid, until the chicken and potatoes are tender.

Serves 4–5
Prep: 15 minutes
Cooking time: 45–55 minutes

pinch of saffron threads
1 chicken stock cube
250ml just-boiled water
8 boneless, skinless chicken thighs
2 preserved lemons (size of a walnut in its shell), rinsed
1 tbsp olive oil
2 medium onions, sliced
3 garlic cloves, finely sliced
1 tsp ground ginger
2 tsp ground cumin
1 tsp paprika
1 tsp dried chilli flakes
2 tbsp cold water
600g medium potatoes, preferably Maris Pipers
3 large ripe tomatoes
50g pitted green olives in brine, drained
20g bunch of fresh coriander, leaves roughly chopped
20g bunch of fresh parsley, leaves roughly chopped
flaked sea salt
freshly ground black pepper

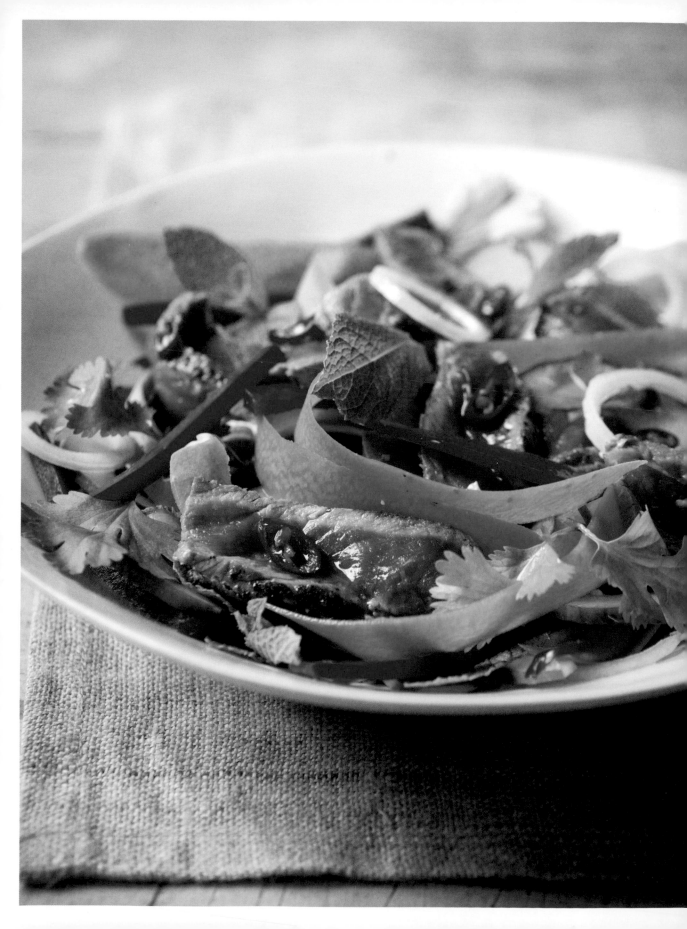

THAI BEEF SALAD

239 calories per portion (if serving 2); 159 calories per portion (if serving 3)

The Kingy and I both love this salad. It's full of fresh, soaring flavours and plenty of heat, but if you don't like your food too spicy, leave out the chilli or deseed it before slicing. Make sure you wash your hands really well after handling the chilli! You can make this with chicken or fish too.

Trim off any visible fat from the steak and season it with salt and lots of freshly ground black pepper. Heat the oil in a small non-stick frying pan and fry the steak over a high heat for 1½ minutes on each side until nicely browned. Leave it to rest on a board while you prepare the veg.

Use a vegetable peeler to peel the carrots into thin ribbons, turning regularly. Cut the cucumber in half lengthways and scoop out the seeds with a teaspoon, then cut the cucumber into slices of about 5mm. Finely slice the shallot. Trim the pepper at both ends and cut it into thin strips. Put all the vegetables in a bowl, then strip the leaves off the herbs, tearing any large leaves in half, and scatter them on top.

To make the dressing, put all the ingredients in a small bowl and whisk until well combined. Cut the steak into slices about 4mm thick and add them to the salad. Pour the dressing over the salad, toss lightly and serve.

Serves 2–3
Prep: 20 minutes
Cooking time: 3 minutes

---

1 lean sirloin or rump steak
  (1.5cm thick)
1 tsp sunflower oil
2 medium carrots, peeled
½ small cucumber
1 long shallot or 2 small shallots,
  trimmed
1 small red pepper, deseeded
25g bunch of fresh coriander
25g bunch of fresh mint
flaked sea salt
freshly ground black pepper

Dressing
1 tbsp nam pla (Thai fish sauce)
1 tbsp light brown soft sugar
1 tbsp fresh lime juice
1 red or green bird's-eye chilli,
  trimmed and very finely sliced

SHREDDED DUCK WRAPS WITH HOISIN SAUCE

131 calories per portion

In our variation of the classic duck dish that everyone loves, we use lettuce instead of pancakes for scooping up the tasty meat. These also make great party canapés or you can take them out for a packed lunch. Just pack all the bits in separate small containers or wrap them in cling film.

Serves 4 (as a light meal or starter)
Prep: 10 minutes
Cooking time: 1 hour

___

2 duck breasts, skin removed
500ml cold water
2 tbsp dark soy sauce
2 star anise
2 garlic cloves, finely sliced
25g chunk of fresh root ginger, peeled and finely sliced
3 spring onions
200g cucumber
2 little gem lettuces
3 tbsp hoisin sauce

Place the skinless duck breasts in a large saucepan and pour the water over them. The duck should be just covered by water so add a little extra if needed. Add the soy sauce, star anise, garlic and ginger and stir well. Bring the liquid to a gentle simmer, cover with a tight-fitting lid and keep at a very gentle simmer for 1 hour. Keep a close eye on it though, and turn the duck halfway through the cooking time.

Just before the duck is ready, prepare the vegetables. Trim the spring onions, cut them in half and slice lengthways. Cut the cucumber into thin matchsticks of about 6cm long. Trim the lettuces, carefully separate the leaves, then wash and drain them well.

After the hour, check that the duck is tender using a fork – the flesh should pull apart easily. Remove the breasts from the cooking liquor and place them on a plate. Discard the cooking liquor.

Shred the duck meat by tearing it apart with 2 forks, then put the duck, cucumber, lettuce, spring onions and sauce on a serving platter or board for sharing.

To eat, place a few strips of cucumber and spring onion on a lettuce leaf and add some warm shredded duck. Spoon over a little hoisin sauce and enjoy.

If you like, you could use Chinese pancakes instead of lettuce, but this will add about 33 calories to each wrap.

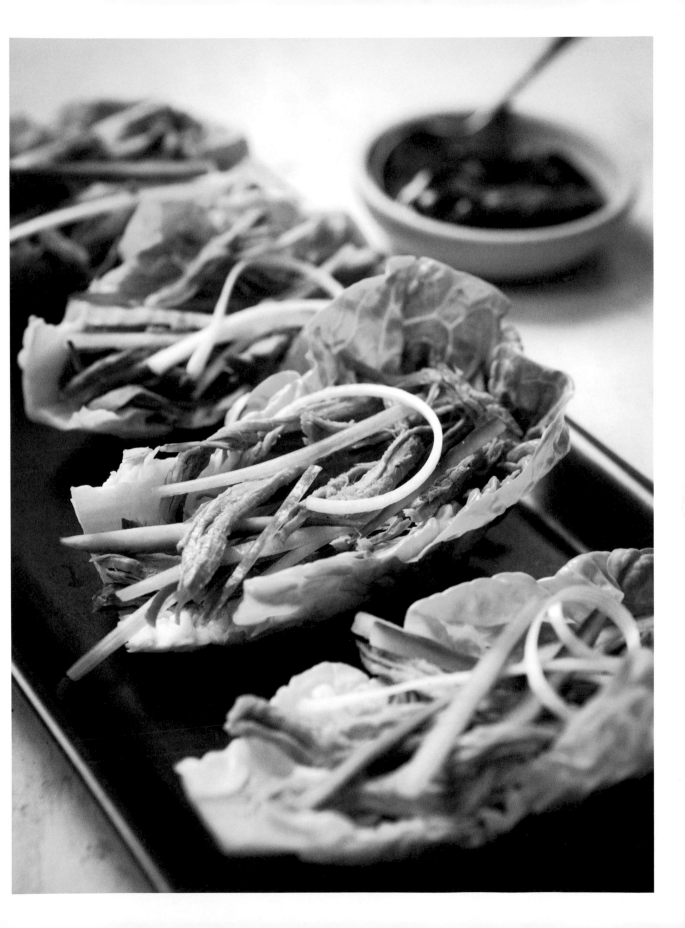

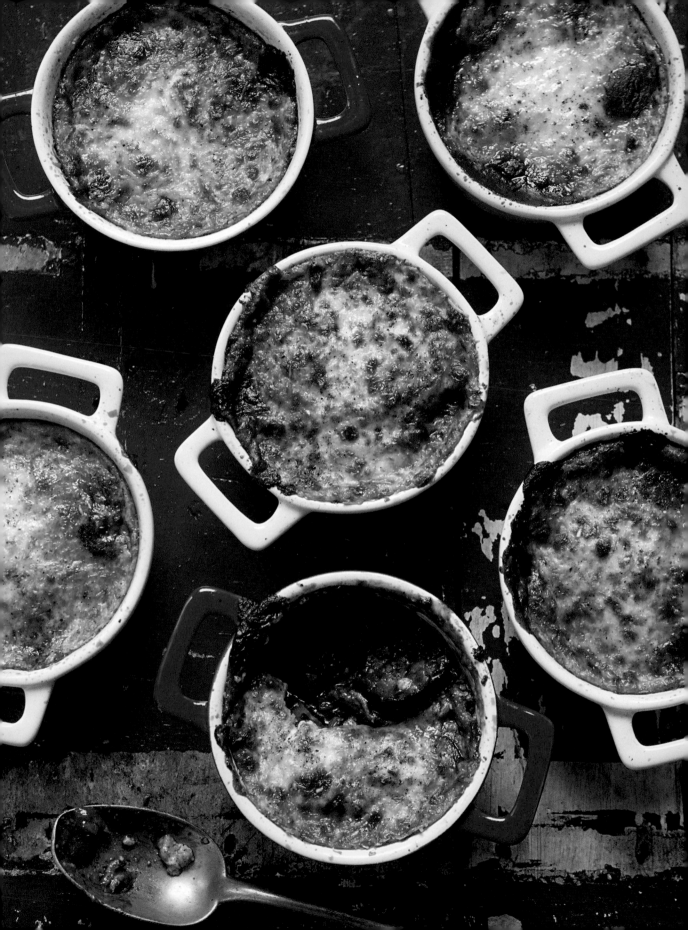

MOUSSAKA

323 calories per portion

Lamb mince can be fatty and high in calories, so look out for lovely lean mince to make these fab little Greek goodies. Our moussakas do look great in individual pots, but you can make them in one big dish if you prefer.

Put the lamb, onion, garlic, oregano, mint, bay leaves and cinnamon in a large non-stick saucepan or sauté pan and cook over a medium heat for 5 minutes. Keep stirring with a wooden spoon to break up the meat.

Stir in the flour and season with salt and plenty of freshly ground black pepper, then add the wine, lamb stock, tomatoes and tomato purée. Bring everything to a simmer, then continue to cook for 10 minutes, stirring occasionally. Add the courgettes and cook for a further 5 minutes until the lamb is tender and the sauce is thick. Remove the bay leaves and cinnamon stick.

Preheat the grill to its hottest setting. Cut the aubergines into 1cm slices, discarding the ends. Arrange the slices in a single layer on a large baking tray, brushing them on both sides with oil. Place the tray under the grill and cook for 5 minutes. Turn the slices over and cook them on the other side for 5 minutes until they're softened and lightly browned. (If you don't have a really big tray, you might need to grill the aubergines in a couple of batches.) Set the aubergines aside.

Preheat the oven to 200°C/Fan 180°C/Gas 6. Just before the mince is ready, make the white sauce. Mix 4 tablespoons of the milk with the cornflour in a small bowl until smooth and put to one side. Pour the rest of the milk into a medium non-stick saucepan and add the bay leaves and half the grated nutmeg. Heat gently for 5 minutes until almost at a simmer, stirring regularly. Remove the bay leaves and whisk in the cornflour mixture, then cook for 3–4 minutes until thickened and smooth, stirring constantly. Remove from the heat and season with salt and lots of freshly ground black pepper.

Spoon a third of the meat sauce into 6 individual ovenproof dishes, then add a layer of aubergines. Repeat the layers twice more, finishing with the aubergines. Pour over the white sauce, making sure it covers in an even layer, then sprinkle with the reserved nutmeg and Parmesan cheese. Bake for 20–25 minutes until the moussakas are golden brown and bubbling.

Serves 6
Prep: 20 minutes
Cooking time: 45 minutes

500g lean lamb mince
1 medium onion, finely chopped
2 garlic cloves, crushed
1½ tsp dried oregano
1 tsp dried mint
2 bay leaves
1 cinnamon stick
2 tbsp plain flour
100ml red wine
400ml lamb stock (made with
    1 lamb stock cube)
400g can of chopped tomatoes
2 tbsp tomato purée
2 medium courgettes, trimmed,
    halved lengthways and sliced
2 medium aubergines (each
    about 275g)
1 tbsp olive oil
flaked sea salt
freshly ground black pepper

White sauce
500ml semi-skimmed milk
4 tbsp cornflour
2 bay leaves
½ tsp freshly grated nutmeg

Topping
20g Parmesan cheese, finely grated

ENCHILADAS

468 calories per portion

A Tex-Mex favourite, this is a dish your whole family will love! You'll need a can of red kidney beans in chilli sauce, which makes a fairly mild chilli mix, but you can add some heat by stirring in some dried chilli flakes before simmering. And if you fancy a bit more heat, you could scatter a few sliced canned jalapeños or finely chopped red chilli over the crème fraiche at the end.

Serves 4
Prep: 20 minutes
Cooking time: 50 minutes

450g extra-lean beef mince
   (5% or less fat)
1 medium onion, chopped
2 garlic cloves, finely chopped
400g can of red kidney beans in
   chilli sauce
3 tbsp tomato purée
½–1 tsp dried chilli flakes (optional)
600ml beef stock, made with
   1 stock cube
oil, for spraying
8 soft corn tortillas
50g half-fat mature Cheddar cheese,
   finely grated
150g half-fat crème fraiche
3 tbsp tomato salsa sauce
   (fresh or from a jar)
fresh coriander, to garnish
lime wedges, to serve
flaked sea salt
freshly ground black pepper

Put a large non-stick frying pan over a medium heat and add the beef, onion and garlic. Cook it all up together for 5 minutes, squishing the mince against the sides of the pan to break it up.

Tip the kidney beans and sauce into the pan and stir in the tomato purée and chilli flakes, if using. Stir in the beef stock and season with a good pinch of salt and plenty of freshly ground black pepper. Bring to a simmer, then reduce the heat and leave to simmer gently for 25–30 minutes, stirring occasionally, until the mince is tender and the sauce has thickened. Stir more regularly towards the end of the cooking time so the sauce doesn't stick. Adjust the seasoning to taste.

Preheat the oven to 200°C/Fan 180°C/Gas 6. Spray a large shallow ovenproof dish with oil or brush it with a little sunflower oil.

Take a tortilla and spoon about an eighth of the mince mixture down the centre. Sprinkle with an eighth of the cheese and fold over one side, then the other and place in the greased dish. Repeat with the remaining tortillas, mince and cheese until everything is used up.

Cover the dish with foil and bake for 15–20 minutes or until the tortillas are piping hot – remove the foil for the last 5 minutes of the cooking time. Spoon the crème fraiche and salsa sauce over the tortillas and garnish with fresh coriander. Season with more black pepper and serve with lime wedges for squeezing.

You can use small flour tortillas if you can't find corn tortillas in your local stores. Don't be tempted to get the large wrap-style tortillas though as they will push the calories up by about 106 per portion.

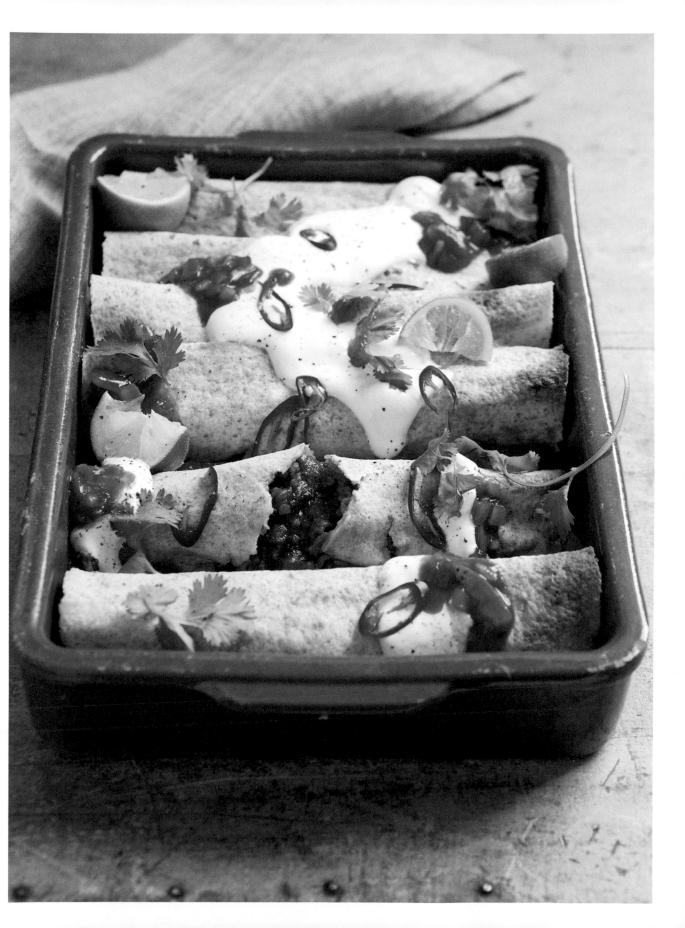

MEALS
ON THE MOVE

"Dieting can be harder when you're on the move. At home, I can make a hearty salad or a bowl of soup for lunch – whatever I fancy. But when I'm out and about or at work it's always a challenge and the temptation is to reach for a sandwich. I never used to look at calorie labels but now I do, and I'm gobsmacked at how those little packets add up – one sandwich can be 500 calories! Not for me any more. Instead, take control of lunchtime and pack your Tupperware with something tasty. When you're tucking into some home-made soup and a wrap, or one of our low-fat Cornish pasties, you'll be the envy of your workmates."

Dave

A BIG SOUP

157 calories per portion

A big soup to make you smaller, this is a tasty wholesome lunch on a cold day. Add a tablespoon of half-fat crème fraiche and a sprinkling of paprika for a guilt-free garnish that adds only 25 calories more per portion.

Serves 6
Prep: 15 minutes
Cooking time: 30 minutes

1 tbsp sunflower oil
1 medium onion, finely sliced
3 garlic cloves, finely sliced
3 medium carrots
150g green beans
75g chorizo sausage, skinned
    and cut into 1cm slices
1 tsp hot smoked paprika
½ tsp flaked sea salt, plus extra
    to season
400g can of chopped tomatoes
1.5 litres chicken stock, fresh
    or made with 1 stock cube
1 tsp caster sugar
400g can cannellini beans, rinsed
    and drained
150g curly kale, thickly shredded
freshly ground black pepper

Heat the oil in a large non-stick saucepan or a big flameproof casserole dish. Add the onion and garlic and fry gently for 5 minutes until softened but not coloured, stirring often. While the onion is frying, peel the carrots and slice them into rough 1.5cm chunks. Trim the green beans and cut them into pieces about 3cm long.

Add the chorizo, paprika and carrots to the pan with the sliced onion and cook over a low heat for 2 minutes, stirring until the chorizo begins to release its fat. Season with salt and lots of black pepper. Tip the tomatoes into the same pan, add the stock and sugar, then turn the heat up to medium.

Bring the liquid to the boil. Reduce the heat slightly and leave the soup to simmer for 12 minutes. Add the canned and fresh beans and the kale and bring it back to a gentle simmer. Cook for 10 minutes until all the vegetables are just tender, adding a little extra water if the soup is looking too thick. Season the soup with salt and black pepper and serve in deep bowls.

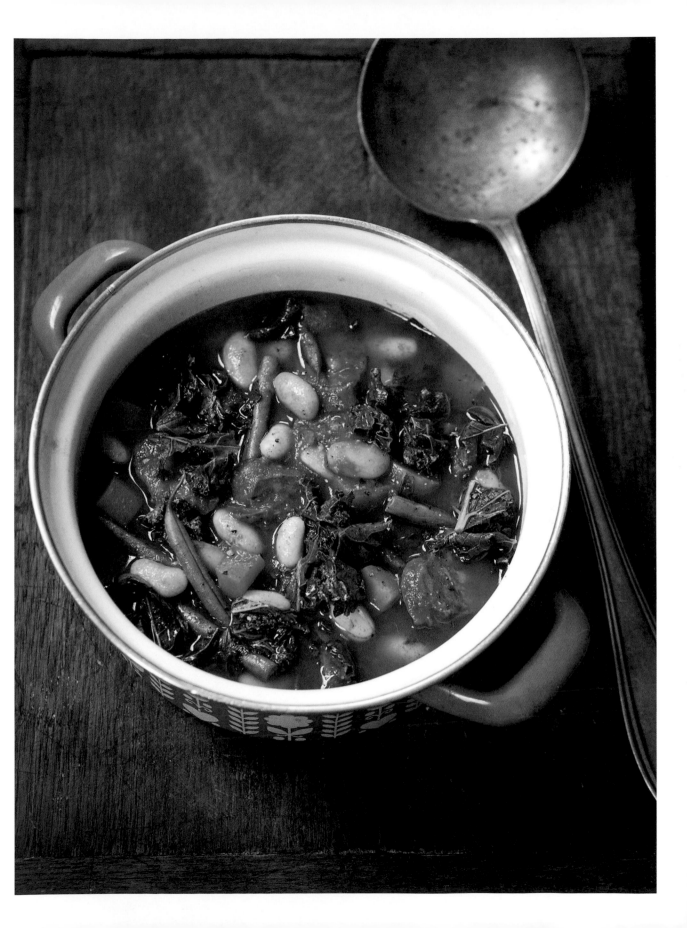

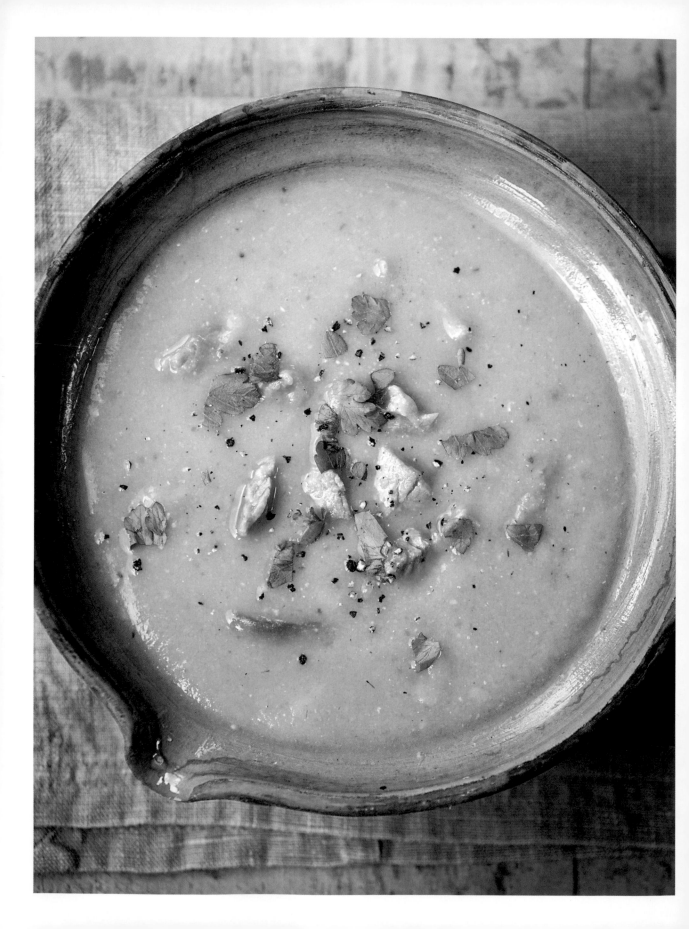

SPLIT PEA SOUP WITH HAM

337 calories per portion (if serving 4); 225 calories per portion (if serving 6)

A dead simple soup that will keep you feeling full for hours, this is another super-healthy reworking of one of our absolute favourites. It takes a little while to cook, but the results are well worth it!

Trim all the fat and rind off the side of the gammon steak and chuck it away. Place the gammon steak in a large saucepan and cover with 2.5 litres of cold water. Add the bay leaf and bring the water to the boil, then skim the surface with a spoon to remove the foam that rises to the top.

Reduce the heat slightly and simmer the gammon for 30 minutes until just tender. Remove the gammon from the water and set it aside on a plate. Leave the water in the pan for cooking the peas.

Rinse the peas in a sieve under cold water, then tip them gently into the pan with the gammon cooking water. Add the chopped onion and thyme and bring it to a gentle simmer, stirring occasionally. Simmer gently for 40 minutes or until the peas are very soft and falling apart. Remove the pan from the heat, pick out the bay leaf and carefully blitz the soup with a stick blender until smooth.

Add the remaining water to the soup until it's the consistency you like. You'll probably need about 500–700ml extra. Tear or chop the gammon into small pieces and add them to the pan. Put the pan back on the heat and bring the soup to a gentle simmer, stirring occasionally. Season to taste and ladle the soup into deep bowls. Sprinkle with some chopped parsley if you like before serving.

Serves 4–6
Prep: 10 minutes
Cooking time: 1 hour and 15 minutes

225g smoked gammon steak
3–3.2 litres cold water
1 bay leaf
300g dried yellow split peas
1 medium onion, roughly chopped
¼ tsp dried thyme
small bunch of flatleaf parsley, chopped, for serving (optional)
flaked sea salt
freshly ground black pepper

CURRIED BUTTERNUT SQUASH AND APPLE SOUP

152 calories per portion

It cheers you up just to look at this soup – it's like a bowl of sunshine. For a veggie-friendly version, use vegetable stock cubes instead of chicken.

Serves 6
Prep: 15 minutes
Cooking time: 40 minutes

1 tbsp sunflower oil
2 medium onions, chopped
1kg butternut squash, peeled, deseeded and cut into 3cm chunks
2 tbsp medium curry powder
2 garlic cloves, crushed
4 eating apples (about 500g), peeled, cored and thickly sliced
1 litre chicken stock, made with 1 stock cube
1 bay leaf
200ml apple juice (preferably pressed/cloudy)
flaked sea salt
freshly ground black pepper

Heat the oil in a large non-stick saucepan, add the onions and cover the pan with a lid. Cook for 5 minutes over a medium-low heat, stirring occasionally. Add the squash, cover the pan again and cook for another 5 minutes until the squash is beginning to soften and brown lightly, stirring once or twice.

Add the curry powder, garlic and apples and cook for 1 minute more, stirring constantly. Pour in the stock, add the bay leaf and bring to the boil. Reduce the heat to a simmer and cook for about 30 minutes or until the squash is very soft, stirring occasionally.

Remove the pan from the heat. Season the soup with salt and pepper and carefully blitz with a stick blender until smooth, or leave it to cool for a while, then blend in a food processor. If you like a extra-smooth soup, pass it through a fine sieve into a clean pan, using the base of a ladle to press the vegetables through the sieve.

Stir the apple juice into the soup, adding a little extra if needed to get the consistency you like, then adjust the seasoning to taste. Reheat gently just before serving, stirring constantly.

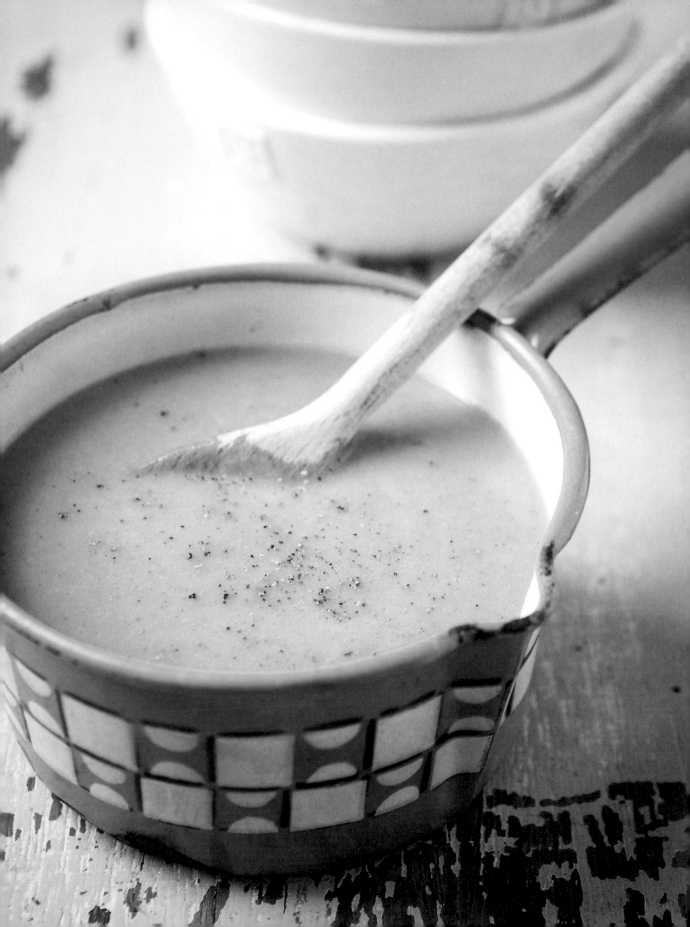

LOW-FAT CORNISH PASTY

396 calories per pasty

The pasty was invented as a convenient way of taking your meal to work and it still is. We've come up with a version that's heavy on carrot, light on potato, and uses a special low-fat pastry. Clever, eh?

Makes 8
Prep: 40 minutes, plus resting time
Cooking time: 50 minutes

1 medium potato (about 125g),
    peeled
200g swede, peeled
1 medium onion, finely chopped
400g beef feather steak or lean
    braising steak, trimmed of hard
    fat or gristle
2 tbsp plain flour
flaked sea salt
freshly ground black pepper

Pastry
500g premium white bread mix
about 320ml lukewarm water
2–3 tbsp plain flour, for rolling
1 medium egg, beaten (to glaze)

Cut the potato and swede into cubes of about 1cm. Put them in a large mixing bowl with the onion and season with a little salt and plenty of ground black pepper. Slice the beef into 5mm strips. Snip them very carefully with kitchen scissors until as finely chopped as possible and put them in a separate bowl. Season with more salt and lots more pepper, then toss with the flour until evenly coated.

For the pastry, place the bread mix in a bowl or food mixer and add the warm water according to the packet instructions. Mix and knead together for 5 minutes to form a ball of dough. Place the dough on a floured surface and leave for 5 minutes. Knead and stretch for 2 minutes more, then form into a ball and leave to rest for 5 minutes.

Roll the dough out on a lightly floured surface until it is about 5mm thick. Using a 15cm side plate or upturned bowl, cut out 8 rounds, re-rolling as necessary.

Mix the vegetables and meat together, then divide the mixture between the pastry rounds, placing the filling on one side and leaving a border of about 2cm. Brush around the edge very lightly with a little water, then bring the empty side over the filling and press the edges together. Roll the edge of the sealed side in on itself once to seal firmly.

Put the pasties on a large baking tray lined with baking parchment. If you want extra-large pasties, cover them loosely with lightly oiled cling film and leave to rise in a warm place for at least 40 minutes or until the dough is looking very puffy; if you are a bit pushed for time, you can bake the pasties right away. Preheat the oven to 180°C/Fan 160°C/Gas 4.

Brush each of the pasties with a little beaten egg to glaze and bake for 15 minutes. Take them out of the oven, cover the pasties with a large sheet of foil, then put them back in the oven for another 30 minutes. Leave to stand at room temperature for 5 minutes before uncovering. Serve warm or cold.

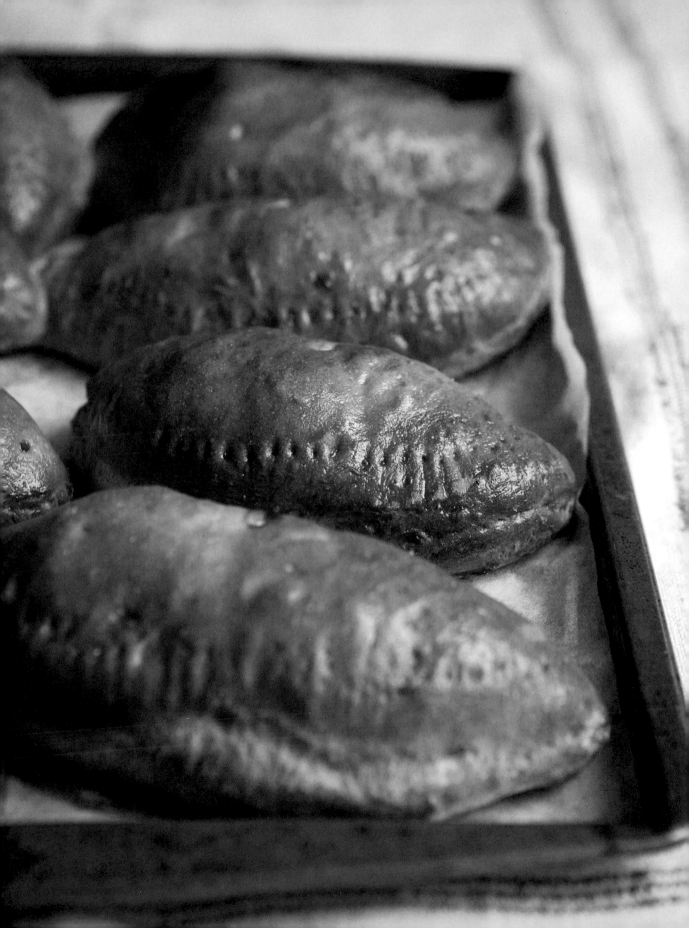

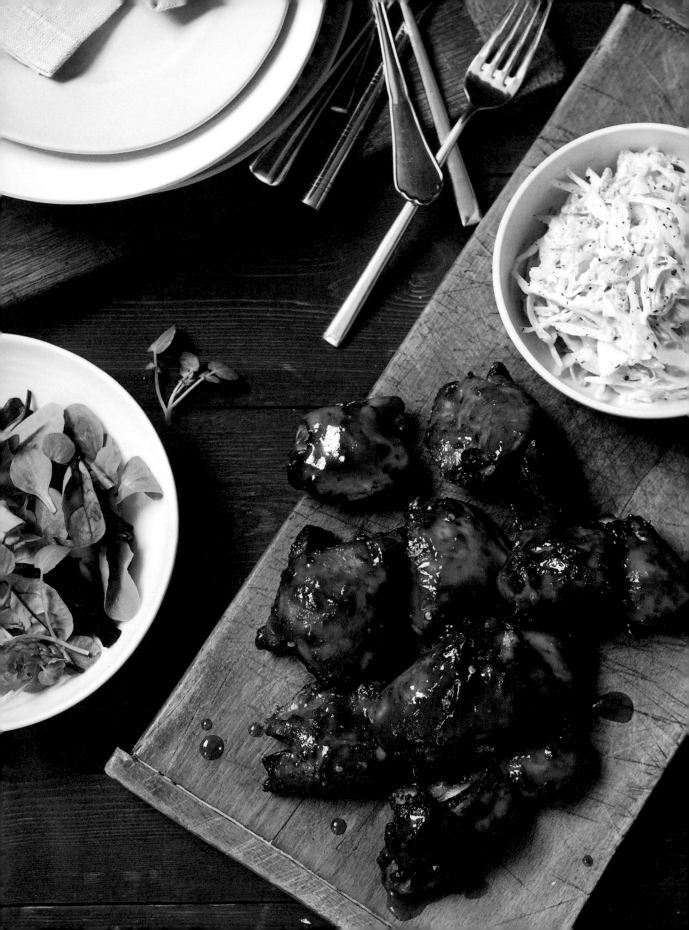

STICKY CHICKEN WITH COLESLAW

320 calories per portion
(chicken thighs: 226 calories per portion; coleslaw: 94 calories per portion)

Make extra of this and serve the chicken hot for supper, then take some to work to eat cold for lunch. We think a lightly dressed green salad goes well, but you could also have a small portion of boiled new potatoes if you like – add an extra 94 calories for a 125g portion of new potatoes.

Preheat the oven to 200°C/Fan 180°C/Gas 6. Line a large baking tray with foil. Place the chicken thighs on a board and carefully trim off as much visible fat as possible with a sharp knife. Season with freshly ground black pepper.

Put the ketchup, vinegar, honey, Worcestershire sauce and dried chilli flakes in a medium non-stick saucepan and bring to a simmer over a low heat, stirring constantly. Remove the pan from the heat and stir in the chicken thighs, turning until they are all thoroughly coated with the sauce. Place them on the baking tray and cook in the oven for 15 minutes.

While the chicken is cooking, remove any damaged leaves from the cabbage and cut out the tough central core. Finely slice the cabbage, separate the leaves and put them in a large bowl. Peel and coarsely grate the carrot and finely slice the spring onions. Add the carrot and spring onions to the cabbage. Spoon the mayonnaise and yoghurt on top and season with lots of freshly ground black pepper. Mix everything together well.

Remove the chicken thighs from the oven and brush them with any of the sauce that has dripped off on to the baking tray. Return to the oven for a further 10 minutes or until the chicken is cooked and the coating is glossy. Serve the chicken hot or cold with the coleslaw and a fresh green salad.

Serves 4
Prep: 10 minutes
Cooking time: 25 minutes

8 boneless, skinless chicken thighs
5 tbsp tomato ketchup
1 tbsp red or white wine vinegar
2 tbsp runny honey
2 tbsp Worcestershire sauce
½ tsp dried chilli flakes (optional)
flaked sea salt
freshly ground black pepper

Coleslaw
¼ white cabbage (about 150g)
1 medium carrot
4 spring onions, trimmed
75g light mayonnaise
125g fat-free natural yoghurt
freshly ground black pepper

HAM SALAD WRAPS

325 calories per wrap

A juicy salad in a wrap makes a lovely generous sandwich without too much stodge, so try our tasty ham wrap or one of the variations below. The wraps can be prepared the night before and stored in the fridge, ready to take to work the next day.

Serves 2

2 large flour tortillas or wraps
   (ideally white and wholemeal
   flour mixed)
1 small romaine lettuce heart,
   trimmed and shredded
1 red pepper, deseeded and cut into
   thin sticks
160g cucumber, cut into thin sticks
1 medium carrot, peeled and
   coarsely shredded
4 slices of good-quality
   wafer-thin ham
2 tbsp ready-made half-fat
   creamy dressing
freshly ground black pepper

Place the tortillas on a board and top them with half the shredded lettuce. Place the pepper and cucumber sticks down the middle of each tortilla, facing them in the same direction. Scatter the carrot over and top with the ham. Drizzle with the dressing, season and top with the rest of the lettuce.

Fold the bottom of each wrap inwards to stop the filling falling out, then roll up fairly tightly and wrap with foil or baking parchment if you're not eating immediately. Chill until needed, but eat within 24 hours. If you're taking these to work for a packed lunch, carry them with an ice pack to keep them cool and fresh.

Tuna and sweetcorn

130g can of tuna in water or brine
198g can of sweetcorn, drained
2 tbsp light mayonnaise
tortillas and salad as above

TUNA AND SWEETCORN WRAPS

343 calories per wrap

Flake the tuna and mix it with the sweetcorn and mayonnaise. Fill the tortillas with lettuce, pepper, cucumber and carrot as above, top with the tuna mixture, then wrap and roll.

Hot-smoked salmon

100g hot-smoked salmon
2 small pickled beetroots, drained
   and sliced
2 gherkins, drained and sliced
2 tbsp light mayonnaise
2 tbsp cold water
tortillas and salad as above

HOT-SMOKED SALMON WRAPS

316 calories per wrap

Flake the salmon and mix it with the sliced beetroots and gherkins. Fill the tortillas with lettuce, pepper, cucumber and carrot as above, then add the salmon mixture. Stir the mayonnaise and the cold water until smooth and drizzle it over the filling, then wrap and roll.

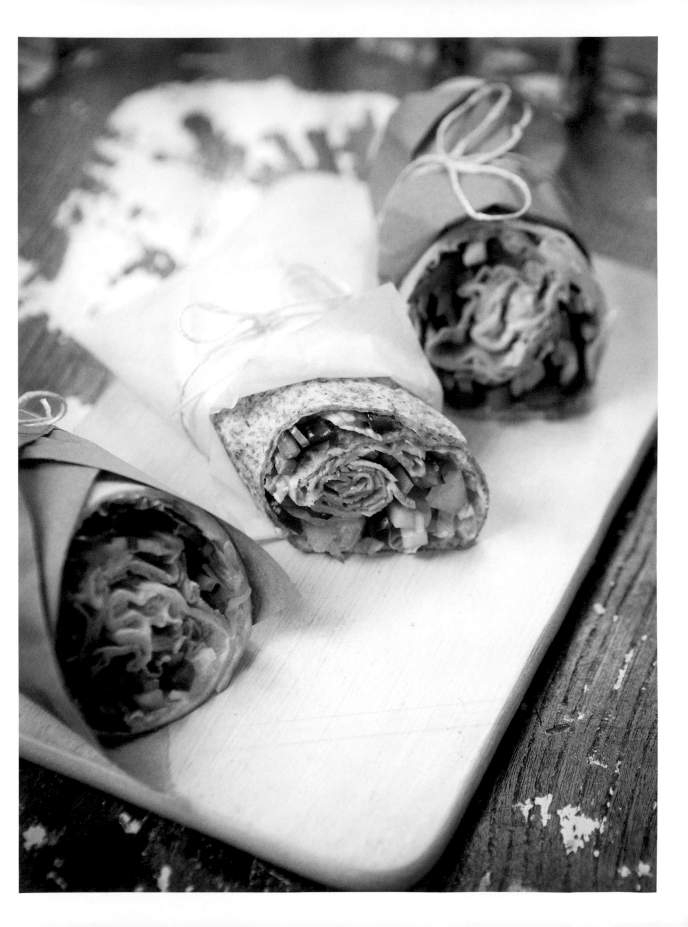

SNACKS AND SALADS

"No longer do I reach for the biscuit barrel when I fancy a little something. It used to be that there was nothing I liked better than a custard cream, but now I'm more likely to go for a punnet of blueberries, a bowl of air-popped popcorn, or some veggie sticks and a tasty dip. Another favourite of mine is gazpacho. You can put it together in minutes and it's great to have in the fridge for when you need something flavour packed and fast. Its spicy goodness fends off the naughty cravings. We also sometimes use a snack to miss a meal. You slake that moment of hunger and next thing you know you've forgotten about lunch. Calories in the bank!"

Si

SWEET AND SAVOURY POPCORN

98 calories per portion with salt; 117 calories per portion with maple syrup;
117 calories per portion with dark chocolate

Serves 4
Prep: 2 minutes
Cooking time: 4–6 minutes

oil, for spraying
75g popping corn (maize)

Flavourings
2 tsp flaked sea salt, or to taste
or
2 tbsp maple syrup
or
15g finely grated plain dark
    chocolate

Mist the inside of a large saucepan with oil. Add the corn and cover the pan with a tight-fitting lid. Place over a medium heat and cook for 4–6 minutes. As soon as you can hear the corn popping, give the pan a good shake. Don't be tempted to take off the lid, as hot popcorn could fly out. Continue cooking until the corn stops popping, shaking the pan regularly while holding the lid in place. If you don't move it around, the corn could burn on the base of the pan.

When the popcorn is done, remove the pan from the heat and tip the kernels into a large bowl, avoiding any that haven't popped. While the popcorn is warm, sprinkle with salt, crushing it between your fingertips, drizzle with maple syrup or sprinkle with grated chocolate. Toss until all the corn is lightly coated and serve warm.

ST CLEMENT'S SQUASH

32 calories per portion (diluted with water)

Makes 750ml (serves 16 when
diluted with water)
Prep: 15 minutes
Cooking time: 5 minutes

3 large lemons, well washed
3 large oranges, well washed
300ml cold water
100g caster sugar
lemon or lime slices, to serve
    (optional)

Peel off the lemon and orange zest with a vegetable peeler, taking care to avoid the white pith. Put the zest in a saucepan. Cut the fruit in half and squeeze the juice. You will need 175ml of lemon juice and 300ml of orange juice to make the squash.

Add the juice, water and sugar to the citrus zest in the pan and place it over a medium heat. Stir regularly until the sugar dissolves, then bring to a simmer and cook for 2 minutes. Remove from the heat and leave to cool. Pour the cooled squash into a clean bottle or jug – you can pour it through a fine sieve first if you like – then cover and chill. It should keep well for 3 days in the fridge.

When ready to serve, pour 3 tablespoons of the squash into a glass and top it up with 200–250ml of chilled fizzy or still water. You can adjust the amount of squash and water to taste, but remember that each tablespoon of squash contains about 10 calories. Add a couple of lemon or lime slices and some ice if you like.

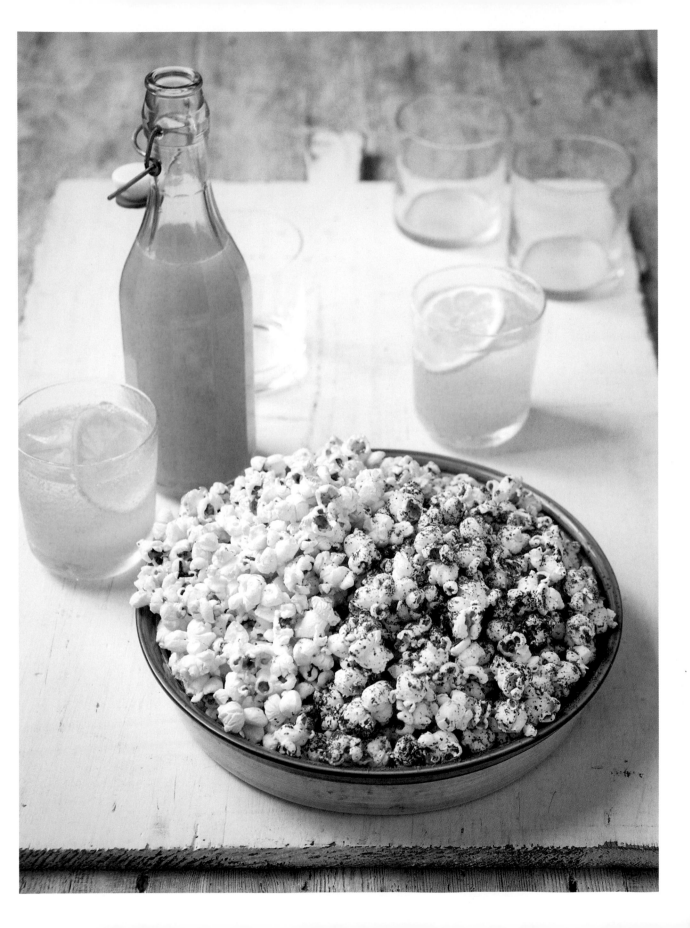

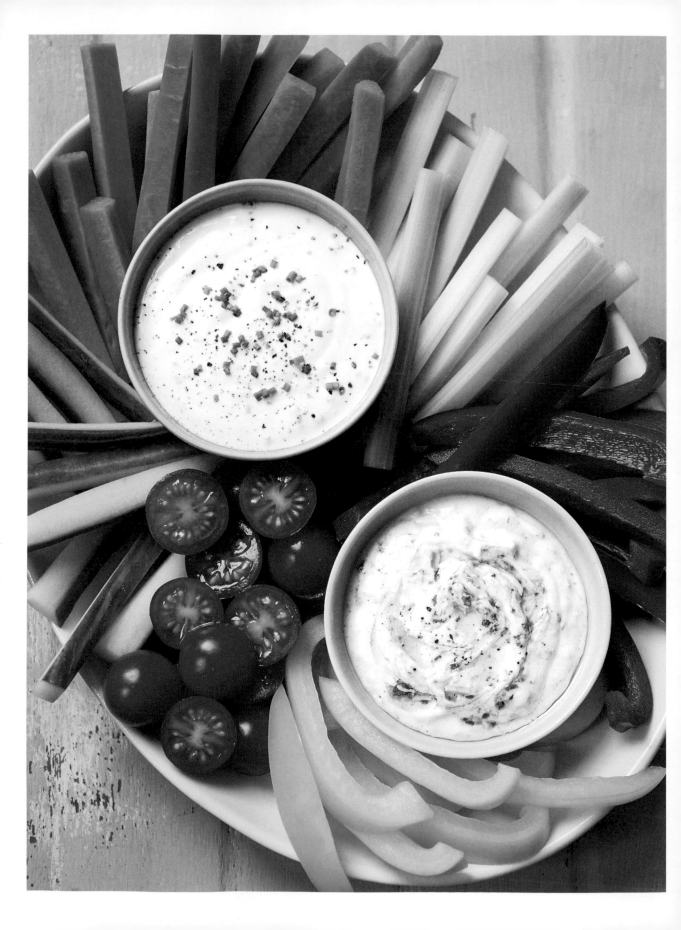

LOVELY DIPS AND STICKS

Take your pick from our choice of delicious dips and serve with colourful vegetable sticks. These are crudités with manners! Great as a snack or something tasty to serve with drinks, and good for packed lunches too.

CRUNCHY VEGETABLE STICKS

31 calories per portion

Deseed the peppers and cut them into wide strips. Trim the celery sticks and cut them into short lengths. Peel the carrots and cut them and the cucumber into wide strips. Cut the tomatoes in half or leave them whole, depending on how big they are. Arrange the veg on a platter and serve with your choice of dip.

Serves 6 with dips
Prep: 10 minutes

1 small red pepper
1 small yellow pepper
2 celery sticks
2 medium carrots
¼ cucumber
150g cherry tomatoes

CREAMY PESTO DIP

62 calories per portion

To make the creamy pesto dip, mix the yoghurt, crème fraiche and pesto sauce in a bowl until well combined.

Serves 6
Prep: 5 minutes

5 tbsp fat-free yoghurt
3 tbsp half-fat crème fraiche
1 tbsp fresh basil pesto sauce

SOURED CREAM AND CHIVE DIP

90 calories per portion

To make the soured cream and chive dip, mix the soured cream, mayonnaise, garlic and chives in a small bowl until well combined.

Serves 6
Prep: 5 minutes

150ml soured cream
1 tbsp light mayonnaise
1 garlic clove, crushed
1 tbsp finely snipped fresh chives

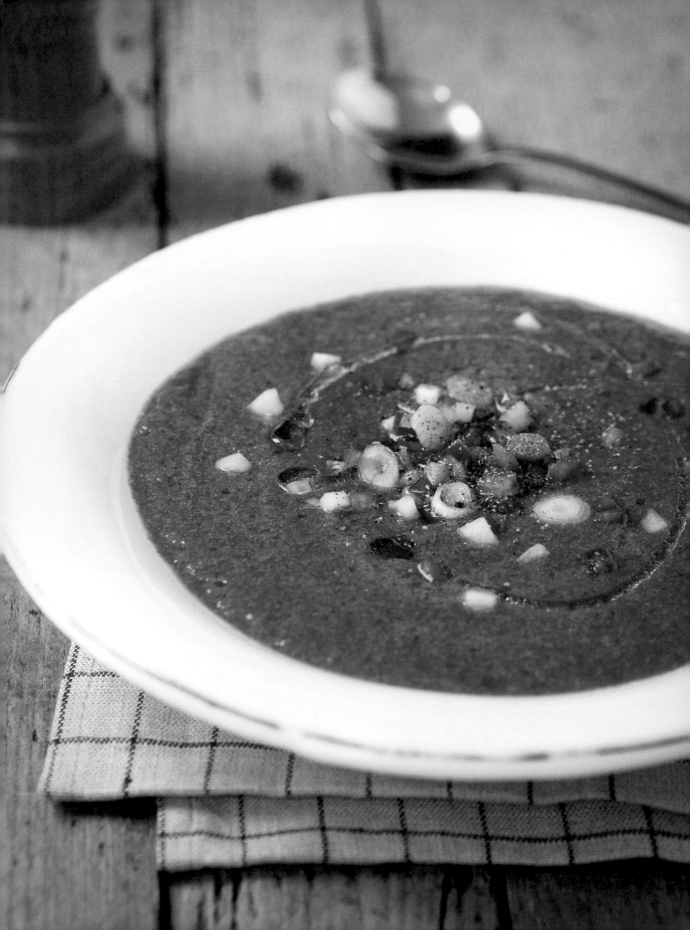

GAZPACHO

71 calories per portion (including oil garnish)

This wonderful Spanish cold soup is great at any time but we love to have a bowlful in the fridge for a guilt-free snack when the cravings get too much! It's refreshing and tastes fantastic.

Make a small, shallow cross in the base of each tomato and place them all in a large heatproof bowl. Pour over enough just-boiled water to cover the tomatoes and leave them to stand for 30–60 seconds. If the tomatoes are ripe enough, the skins should loosen and wrinkle back.

Remove the tomatoes with a slotted spoon and when they're cool enough to handle, peel off the skins. Cut out the tough central core and dice the rest of the flesh, then put all but a couple of tablespoons of the diced tomatoes in a food processor. Set aside the rest in a bowl.

Cut the peppers into quarters and remove the seeds. Cut a quarter of each pepper into small dice and add these to the bowl with the diced tomatoes. Roughly chop the remaining pepper quarters and put them in the food processor. Peel the cucumber and cut it in half lengthways, then scoop out the seeds. Cut about a quarter of the peeled cucumber into small dice and add this to the diced tomatoes and peppers. Roughly chop the rest and put it in the food processor.

Trim and finely slice 2 of the spring onions and add them to the diced vegetables, then cover the bowl with cling film and put it in the fridge. Trim and roughly chop the remaining spring onions and add them to the food processor.

Peel and roughly chop the garlic and scatter it over the veg in the food processor. Pour over the tomato juice and add 2 tablespoons of the red wine vinegar, the salt and lots of ground black pepper. Blitz until as finely blended as possible. Taste the soup and add more vinegar, salt and pepper if needed – you want your gazpacho to be pretty punchy. Whizz again, then tip it all into a bowl, cover and chill for a couple of hours before serving.

Ladle into deep bowls and top with the diced vegetables. Season with a little more black pepper, drizzle each serving with a little olive oil if you like and serve. (If you don't have time to chill the gazpacho, add a couple of ice cubes to each bowl.)

Serves 6
Prep: 20 minutes

400g fresh, ripe tomatoes (about 4)
1 green pepper
1 red pepper
½ large cucumber
1 bunch of spring onions (about 10)
2 garlic cloves
1 litre tomato juice, well chilled
2–3 tbsp red wine vinegar
3 tsp extra virgin olive oil (optional)
1½ tsp flaked sea salt
freshly ground black pepper
ice cubes, to serve (optional)

ASPARAGUS WRAPPED IN PARMA HAM

100 calories per portion with basil dip
113 calories per portion baked with Parmesan

When asparagus is in season it makes a perfect snack or starter, especially when wrapped in delicious Parma ham. Serve hot or cold, depending on what you fancy!

Serves 4
Prep: 10 minutes
Cooking time: 2–10 minutes

250g bunch of asparagus
   (about 14 spears)
80g packet of Parma ham
   (7–8 slices)

Creamy basil dip
2 tbsp half-fat crème fraiche
2 tbsp light mayonnaise
1 tsp fresh lemon juice
1 tsp fresh basil pesto sauce

Baked with Parmesan
3 tbsp half-fat crème fraiche
10g Parmesan cheese, finely grated

Half fill a large frying pan with water and bring it to the boil. Snap off the woody ends of the asparagus spears. Add the asparagus to the boiling water and return to the boil, then cook for 1–2 minutes according to the thickness of the spears.

Immediately drain the asparagus in a colander and rinse it under plenty of running water until completely cold. The asparagus should still be quite crisp. Tip it on to a board.

Cut the slices of Parma ham in half and wrap each of the asparagus spears in a piece of ham.

To serve cold with the dip, arrange the wrapped asparagus on a serving plate. Mix the crème fraiche with the mayonnaise, lemon juice and pesto. Spoon into a small dish and serve with the asparagus for dipping.

To serve hot, put the wrapped asparagus in a shallow ovenproof dish, then dot with teaspoons of the crème fraiche and sprinkle with Parmesan. Bake in a preheated oven at 200°C/Fan 180°C/Gas 6 for about 15 minutes until hot and lightly browned. Alternatively, arrange the spears in a single layer on a baking tray and brown them under the grill for 5–6 minutes.

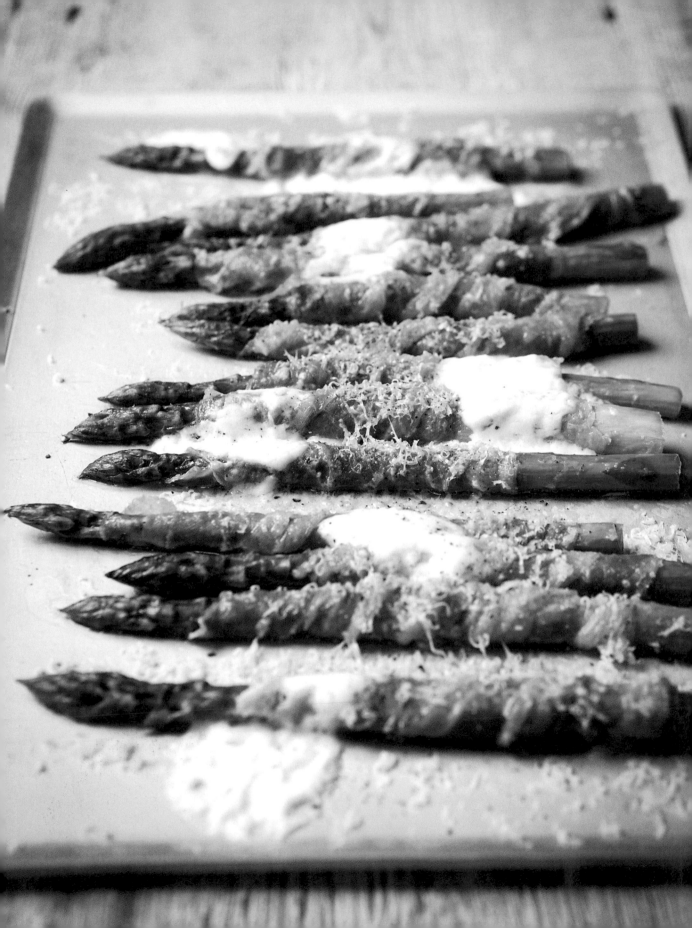

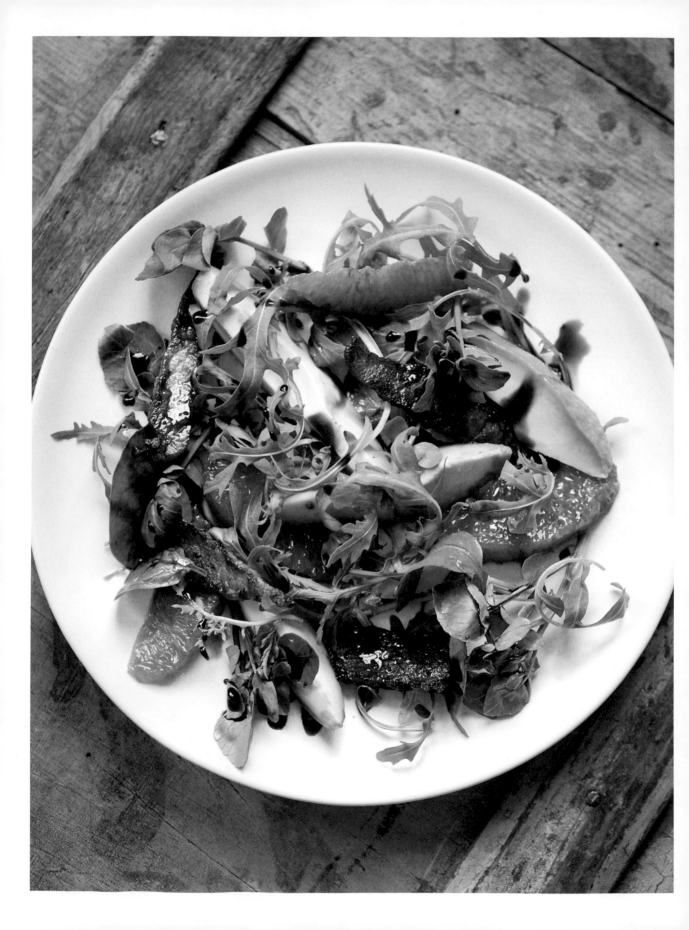

GRAPEFRUIT, AVOCADO AND BACON SALAD

154 calories per portion

Fresh and tangy with that lovely bacon crunch, this is one of our favourite salads and something we're always happy to eat.

Place the grapefruit on a chopping board and slice off the top and bottom with a sharp knife. Rest the fruit on one of the cut ends and cut off the peel and pith, working your way around the grapefruit.

Next, cut between the membranes to release the segments. Put the segments in a salad bowl together with any juice that's on your board.

Remove the stone from the avocado and use a large spoon to ease the flesh from the skin. Put the avocado flesh on a board and cut it into slices. Put the salad leaves in a bowl and toss them lightly with the grapefruit segments and avocado.

Trim any visible fat off the bacon rashers and cut them into 2cm-wide strips. Heat the oil in a small non-stick frying pan over a medium heat and fry the bacon strips in the hot pan for 3–4 minutes until lightly browned.

Take the pan off the heat and scatter the bacon over the salad. Add the water and balsamic vinegar to the hot frying pan and stir until combined, then drizzle over the salad. Serve immediately.

Serves 2
Prep: 10 minutes
Cooking time: 3–4 minutes

---

1 ruby or pink grapefruit
½ ripe but firm avocado
2 large handfuls of watercress, spinach and rocket salad
2 rashers of rindless smoked back bacon
2 tsp olive oil
1 tbsp cold water
2 tsp good balsamic vinegar

CHICKPEA, HOT-SMOKED SALMON AND POMEGRANATE SALAD

222 calories per portion

With a rich mix of pulses and smoked fish, this is a really satisfying salad – luscious and crunchy with a hint of spice. Looks and tastes a million dollars and makes a good packed lunch too.

Serves 4
Prep: 10 minutes

1 pomegranate
½ cucumber
400g can of chickpeas, rinsed
    and drained
¼ medium red onion, finely sliced
2 ripe tomatoes, each cut into
    12 chunks
15g bunch of fresh coriander,
    leaves roughly chopped
20g bunch of flatleaf parsley,
    leaves roughly chopped
150g skinless, hot-smoked salmon
    or trout

Dressing
1 tsp runny honey
1 tsp harissa paste
2 tsp fresh lemon juice
1 tbsp extra virgin olive oil
flaked sea salt
freshly ground black pepper

Cut the pomegranate in half. Hold each half over a bowl and bash the back with a wooden spoon to dislodge the seeds – you may need to help some of them out with a knife or spoon. Put the seeds and any juice in a serving bowl. Peel the cucumber in long strips, leaving a little skin between each strip, then quarter lengthways and cut into 1.5cm slices.

Tip the chickpeas into the bowl, add the onion, tomatoes, cucumber, coriander and parsley and mix well. Flake the fish into chunks on top of the salad.

To make the dressing, put the honey, harissa and lemon juice in a small bowl and whisk with a small metal whisk or a fork to combine. Add the olive oil, season with salt and ground black pepper and whisk until thickened. Spoon over the salad and toss lightly to serve. Keeps well in the fridge for a couple of days.

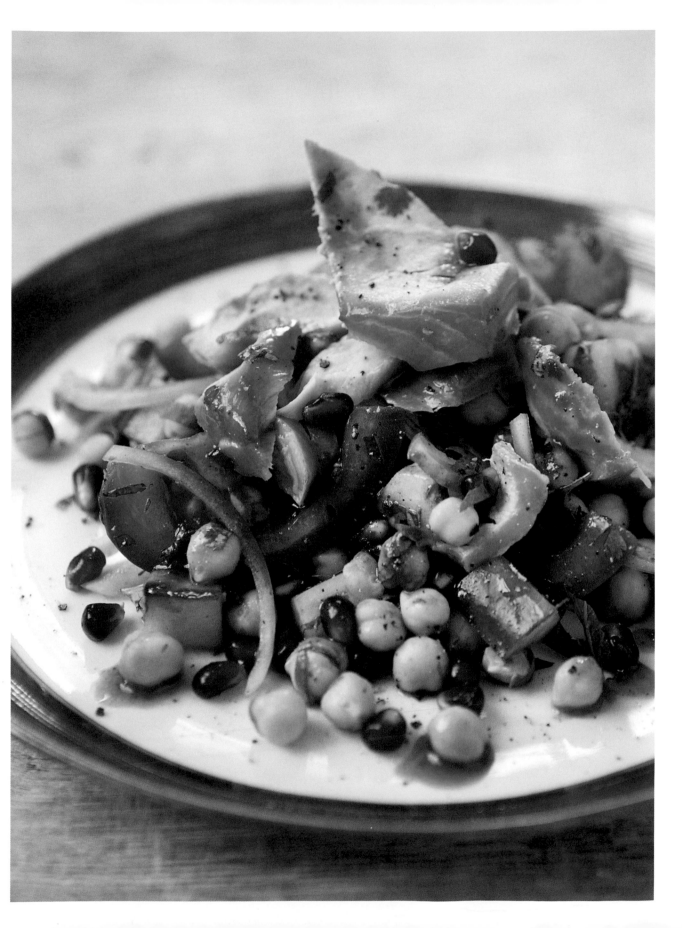

TUNA SALAD WITH RED ONION AND BEANS

161 calories per portion

This is our take on the Italian classic tonno e fagioli, otherwise known as tuna and beans. Every dieter should have a can or two of tuna in the cupboard so you'll know you'll never want for a satisfying snack. Red onions and olives make this extra tasty.

Serves 4
Prep: 15 minutes

1 small red onion

400g can of cannellini beans, rinsed and drained

250g cherry tomatoes, halved

½ cucumber, halved lengthways and sliced

20g bunch of flatleaf parsley, leaves roughly chopped

130g can of tuna steak in water or brine, drained

2 little gem lettuces, leaves separated

50g good black olives in brine, drained and pitted

Dressing
1 garlic clove, crushed
1 tsp caster sugar
1 tsp Dijon mustard
1 tbsp white wine vinegar
1 tbsp cold water
1 tbsp extra virgin olive oil
flaked sea salt
freshly ground black pepper

To make the dressing, put the garlic, sugar, mustard, vinegar and water in a bowl. Season with a pinch of salt and ground black pepper. Whisk with a small metal whisk until well combined. Slowly add the oil, whisking constantly until the dressing is pale and frothy.

Peel the onion and slice it into very thin rings. Put three quarters of the rings in a large serving bowl and add the beans, cherry tomatoes, cucumber, parsley and half the dressing. Toss lightly together, then add the tuna and toss again. You don't want the tuna broken up too much but it should be fairly evenly distributed through the salad.

Line a serving platter with little gem lettuce leaves and spoon the tuna and bean salad on top. Scatter with the remaining onion rings and dot with the pitted olives. Spoon over the rest of the dressing, season with more ground black pepper and serve.

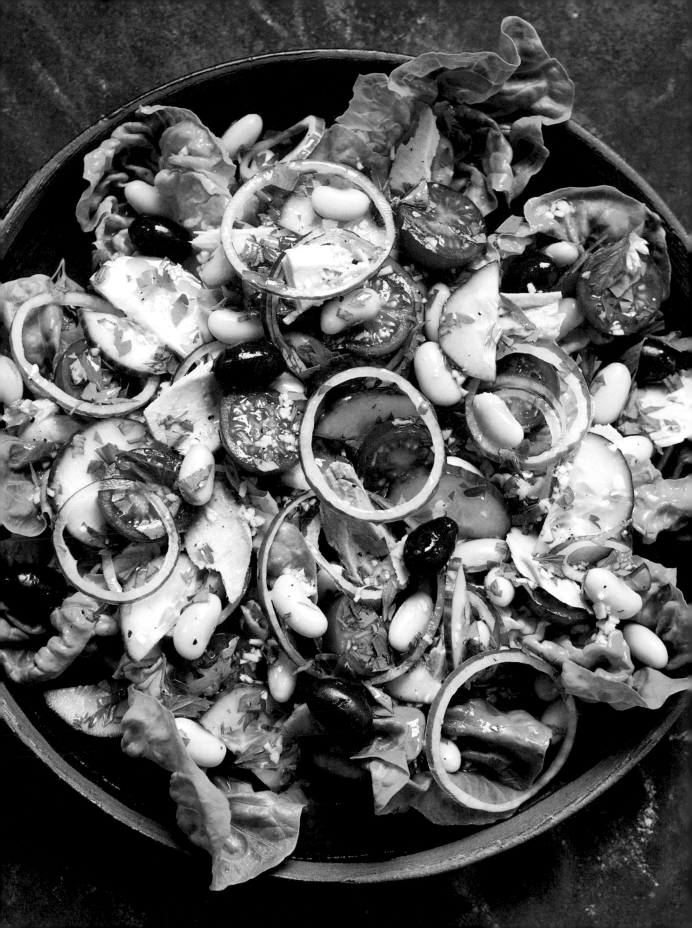

SOMETHING
SWEET

"We all need something sweet once in a while and we've worked out some ways of satisfying a sweet tooth without messing up the diet. Would you believe that even an innocent little humbug is about 35 calories? Our sweet treats are relatively guilt-free but still indulgent. Don't forget that calorie counting is not just about lowering fat but sugar as well. We've made these puds and cakes with as little as possible, relying on the lovely flavour of fruit to supply that hit of sweetness. "

Dave

FRESH FRUIT TRIFLES

239 calories per portion

These stunning little puds are a doddle to make and feel like a real treat. No one will guess that they contain under 250 calories per portion – a sensation on the lips but a mere trifle on the hips.

Serves 6
Prep: 15 minutes,
plus setting time

12 sponge fingers (about 75g)
3 tbsp sweet sherry (optional)
2 x sachets (23g) of raspberry
   flavour sugar-free jelly crystals
300ml just-boiled water
600ml cold water
200g fresh strawberries
300ml low-fat ready-made custard,
   preferably fresh
125ml double cream
100g fresh raspberries
100g fresh blueberries
fresh mint leaves, to decorate

You'll need 6 glass dessert dishes for this; each one needs to hold about 250ml. You can also make the trifle in a large bowl, but it will take a little longer to set. Break the sponge fingers in half and place them in the base of each dish. Drizzle with a little sherry if you like.

Dissolve the jelly crystals in 300ml just-boiled water in a large jug according to the packet instructions. As soon as they have dissolved, stir in the 600ml of cold water.

Hull the strawberries and cut them in half or into quarters if they are very large. Scatter the strawberries over the sponge fingers. Pour the jelly slowly over the broken sponge fingers and strawberries until they are evenly covered. Cover the dishes with cling film and chill in the fridge for 3–4 hours or until the jellies are set.

Take the dishes out of the fridge and remove the cling film. Spoon the custard on top of each jelly without taking it right to the sides.

Put the cream in a bowl and whisk with electric beaters until soft peaks form. Try not to overwhip the cream – it's ready when it looks like soft, billowing clouds. Add a large spoonful of the whipped cream to each trifle, placing it on top of the custard. Decorate the trifles with fresh raspberries, blueberries and a few fresh mint leaves.

These keep well in the fridge so you can make them up to 2 days before serving – ideal if you're planning a party.

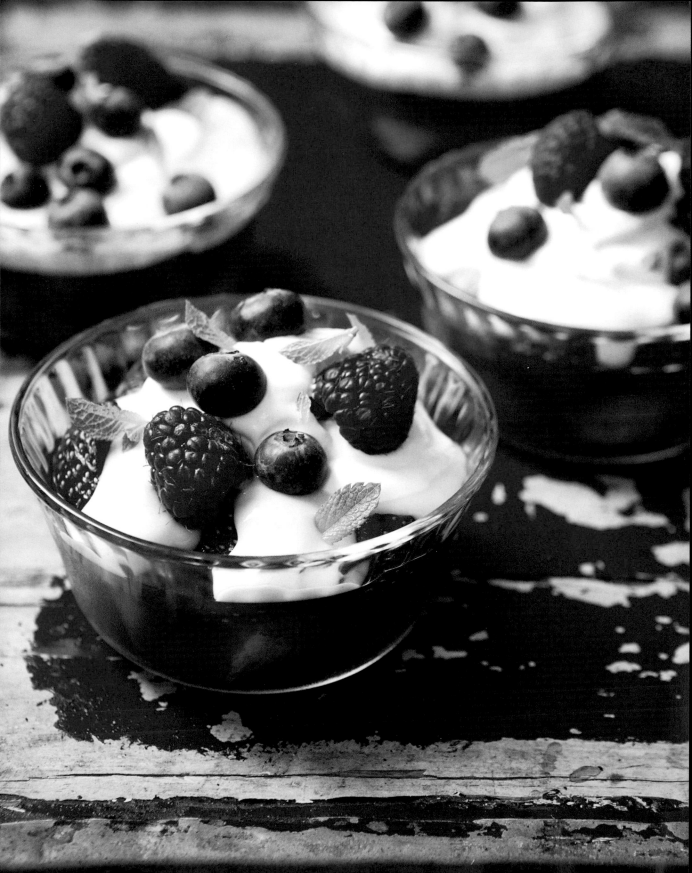

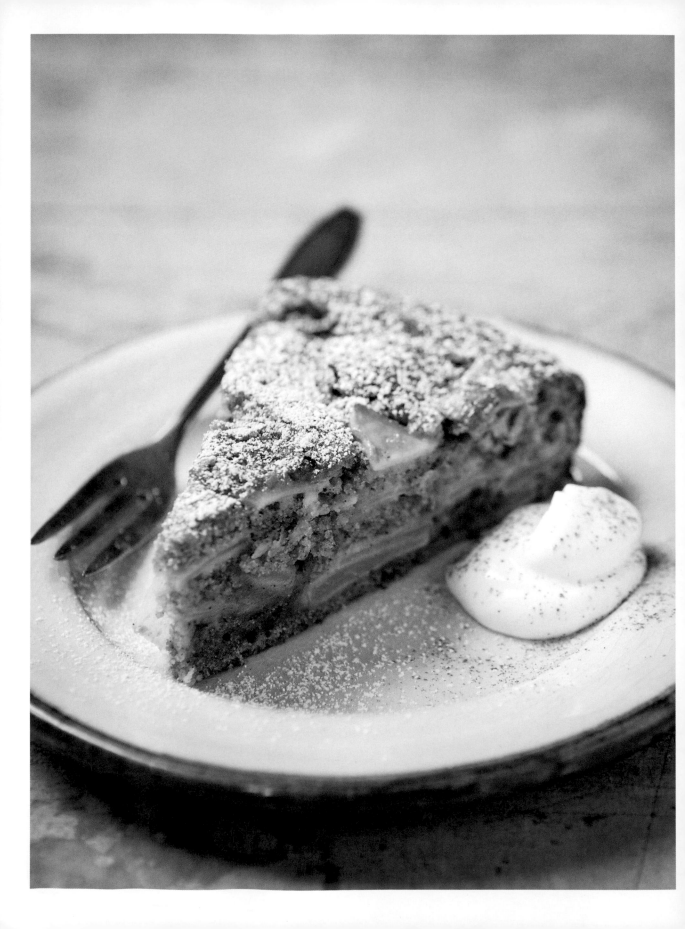

SPICED APPLE CAKE

229 calories per portion (if serving 12); 196 calories per portion (if serving14)

When you're in need of a nice piece of cake to go with a cup of tea this will do the trick. Spiced up with cinnamon and lemon zest it's a fruity delight. Bet you didn't think you could enjoy something like this while on a diet!

Preheat the oven to 190°C/Fan 170°C/Gas 5. Line a 23cm springclip cake tin with baking parchment. Mist the base and sides with oil.

Peel the apples and cut them into quarters. Remove the cores and cut the apples into thin slices – you'll need about 500g prepared weight. Put the apple slices in a bowl and toss with the lemon juice and zest.

Mix the flour, baking powder, cinnamon and spice in a large mixing bowl. Whisk the eggs with the 100g of sugar, the milk and sunflower oil in a separate medium bowl using a large metal whisk. Then pour the wet ingredients into the dry ingredients, stirring lightly until combined – use the whisk to break up any stubborn lumps. Toss the lemony apples through the cake batter until evenly mixed and pour the mixture into the prepared tin.

Sprinkle the 2 tablespoons of sugar evenly over the top and bake the cake in the centre of the oven for 1 hour until it is well risen and golden on top. Test the cake by inserting a skewer into the centre – it should slide easily through the apples in the middle and come out clean.

Leave the cake to cool for 10 minutes before removing it from the tin and carefully peeling off the baking parchment. Dust with sifted icing sugar and serve warm or cold with a little single cream or half-fat crème fraiche.

This cake is deliciously moist, so it's best to keep it wrapped in foil and eat it within a couple of days. It is quite large, so if you want to keep yourself from being tempted to eat too much, you could cut the cake into quarters and freeze some for another time. Wrapped tightly, it will freeze well for 3 months. Defrost the cake fully before serving and warm it through in a low oven or a microwave if you like.

Serves 12–14
Prep: 15 minutes
Cooking time: 1 hour

_____

oil, for spraying
750g Bramley cooking apples
1 tbsp fresh lemon juice
finely grated zest of ½ lemon
250g self-raising flour
1 tsp baking powder
1 tsp ground cinnamon
1 tsp ground mixed spice
2 large eggs
100g demerara sugar, plus 2 tbsp
200ml semi-skimmed milk
100ml sunflower oil
½ tsp sifted icing sugar, for dusting

VERY BERRY FOOL

234 calories per portion

Fruit fools are usually laden with cream but, clever clogs that we are, we've replaced more than half the cream with low-fat custard. Result – that rich texture with fewer cals.

Serves 6
Prep: 10 minutes
Cooking time: 15 minutes, plus chilling time

450–500g frozen mixed berries
200ml double cream, well chilled
300ml low-fat ready-made custard, preferably fresh
fresh mint leaves, to decorate

Put the frozen fruit in a medium non-stick saucepan and heat gently for 5 minutes, stirring occasionally until the berries begin to soften and release their juice. Increase the heat and simmer the fruit very gently for 10 minutes, stirring regularly until very soft and pulpy.

Remove the pan from the heat and press the berries and juice through a sieve over a bowl, using the bottom of a ladle to help you extract as much of the purée as possible. Leave the purée to cool and chuck out the seeds left in the sieve. You should end up with about 175ml of fruit purée.

Whip the cream with an electric whisk until stiff peaks form – don't overwhip, though, or the cream could separate. Pour the custard into a large bowl and whisk in the whipped cream. Stir in three quarters of the berry purée until well combined. Pour the remaining berry purée over the top of the custard mixture and stir once until very lightly combined.

Spoon the fool into individual glass dishes or tumblers – or small wine glasses. It should look quite marbled, so don't stir it too much. Scatter a few tiny mint leaves on top, cover and chill for at least 30 minutes before serving.

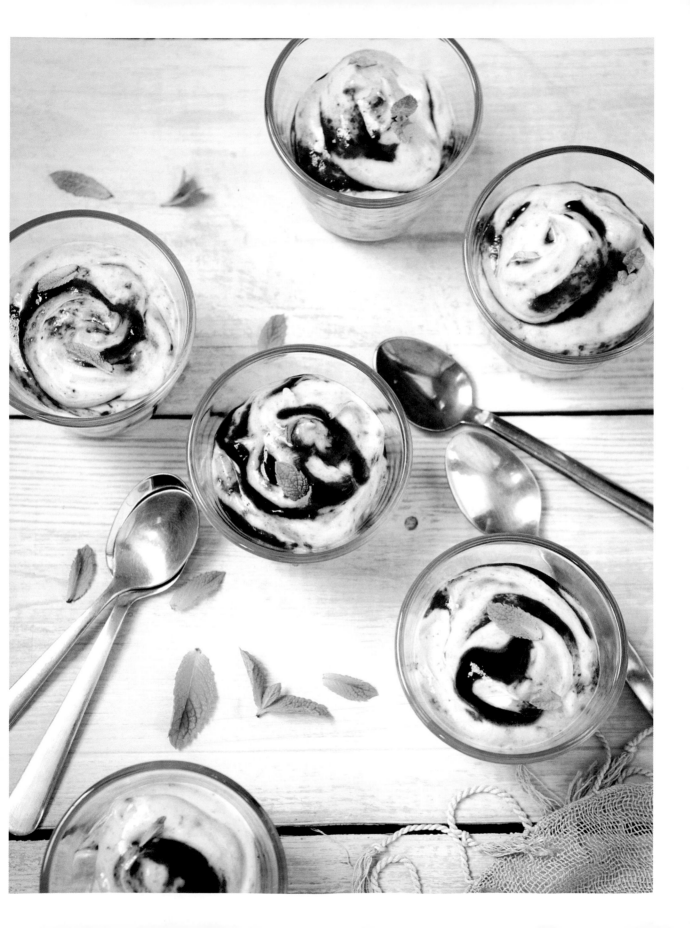

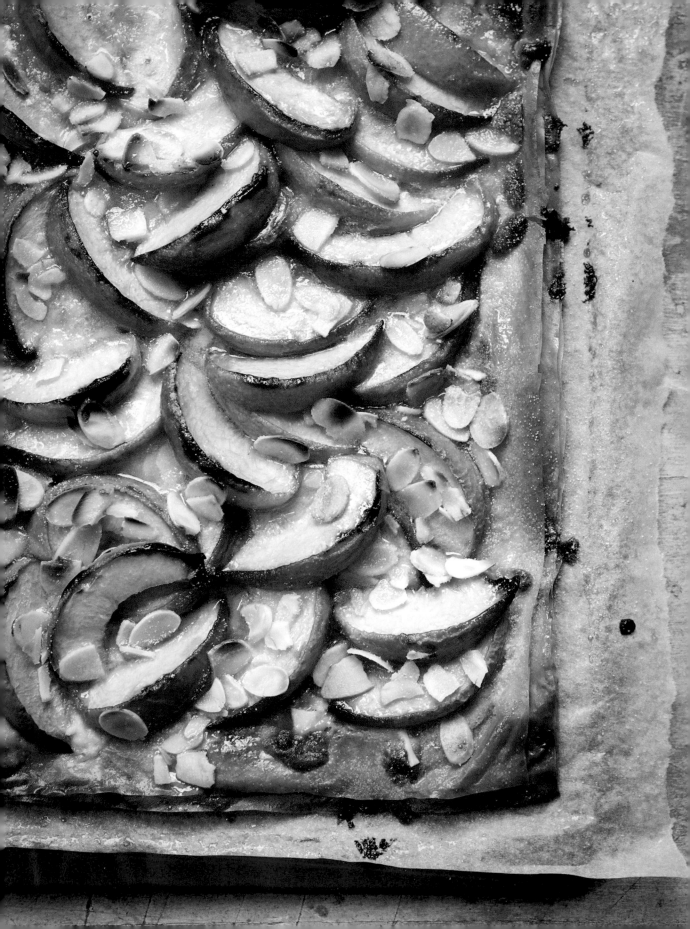

WARM NECTARINE TART

173 calories per portion

Possibly the fastest tart you'll ever make. Topped with a fresh nectarines and a grating of marzipan, this is sweet, succulent and very scrumptious.

Preheat the oven to 190°C/Fan 170°C/Gas 5. Take a nectarine and, holding it carefully, cut out slices from top to bottom towards the stone with a small knife, working your way around the whole fruit. Drop the pieces into a bowl. Slice the rest of the nectarines in the same way – each one should give you 12 slices – and chuck the stones away.

Unroll the filo pastry and cut 2 sheets in half to make 4 squares. Place a square of pastry on a large baking tray that you've lined with baking parchment.

Mist the pastry with oil and cover it with a second square. Repeat the layers of filo twice more until you have a stack of 4 sheets of pastry on the baking tray. Give it another quick spritz with the oil over the top.

Coarsely grate the marzipan over the pastry – taking care not to grate your fingers! Tumble the nectarine slices over the marzipan, leaving a 2cm border all around the edge. Scatter the almonds on top and sprinkle with the sugar.

Bake for 20 minutes or until the fruit is soft and glossy and the pastry is golden brown and crisp. Cut into 4 and serve with half-fat crème fraiche if you like – add 25 calories for each tablespoon.

Serves 4
Prep: 10 minutes
Cooking time: 20 minutes

3 ripe but firm nectarines or peaches
2 sheets of filo pastry, each about
    48 x 25cm
oil, for spraying
50g white or golden marzipan
1 tbsp flaked almonds
2 tsp caster sugar
half-fat crème fraiche (optional)

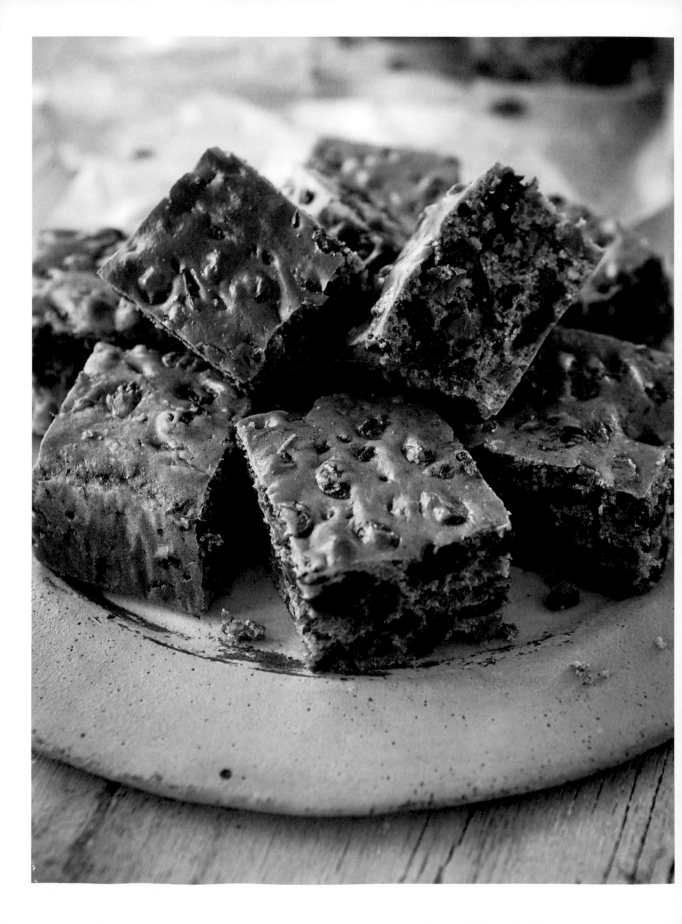

LOW-FAT FRUIT TEA LOAF

157 calories per square

A real tea-time treat. No one will believe that this has no added fat or sugar – it simply tastes too good! Make sure you stick to our recommended serving size, though, and don't be tempted to eat more.

Put the teabag in a jug and add 400ml just-boiled water. Stir and leave to steep for 5 minutes. Finely grate the lemon zest and squeeze the juice, then pour the juice into a large saucepan. Squeeze the teabag and chuck it away, then pour the tea into the pan with the juice. Add the lemon zest, prunes, mixed dried fruit and spice.

Stir well and place the pan over a low heat. Bring to a gentle simmer and cook gently for 5 minutes or until the liquid is almost all absorbed, stirring occasionally. Remove from the heat, tip the mixture carefully into a large mixing bowl and leave to cool for 40 minutes.

Preheat the oven to 170°C/Fan 150°C/Gas 3 1/2. Line the base and sides of a 20 x 30cm rectangular cake tin with baking parchment or use a small roasting tin or a 25cm square cake tin. Peel the banana and cut it into thick slices. Put these in a food processor, add the eggs and milk, then blend to make a purée. Add the flour and baking powder and blend again until smooth.

Pour the egg and banana mixture on to the soaked fruit and stir until thoroughly combined. Spoon the mixture into the prepared tin and level the surface with the back of a spoon. Bake in the centre of the oven for 30 minutes or until the cake is pale golden brown and a skewer inserted into the centre comes out clean. Remove the cake from the oven and cool in the tin for 30 minutes.

Carefully turn the cake out, peel off the baking parchment and leave to cool on a wire rack. When the cake is cool, cut it into 20 squares. Wrap well, store in the fridge and eat within a week.

Cuts into 20 squares
Prep: 15 minutes, plus cooling time
Cooking time: 30 minutes

1 teabag
400ml just-boiled water
1 unwaxed lemon
250g ready-to-eat prunes, quartered
500g luxury dried mixed fruit
3 tsp ground mixed spice
1 ripe medium banana (about 115g peeled weight)
4 large eggs
4 tbsp skimmed milk
300g self-raising flour
½ tsp baking powder

LIGHT CHOCOLATE MOUSSE WITH RASPBERRIES

147 calories per portion

Everyone needs some chocolate from time to time so we had to come up with a chocolate pud for this book. We're happy with this one – see what you think. It's a little indulgence from us to you with our love and has mercifully few calories!

Serves 6
Prep: 10 minutes, plus cooling and chilling
Cooking time: 5 minutes

100g plain dark chocolate (70% cocoa solids)
300g low-fat ready-made custard, preferably fresh
3 large egg whites
150g fresh raspberries
½ tsp icing sugar

To make the mousse, break 95g of the plain chocolate into pieces and place these in a large heatproof bowl. Set the bowl over a pan of gently simmering water until almost melted.

Remove the bowl carefully from the pan and stir the chocolate with a wooden spoon until it's smooth. Leave to cool for about 15 minutes but don't let the chocolate set.

Stir the custard into the melted chocolate until smooth. Whisk the egg whites in a large bowl with an electric whisk until fairly stiff but not dry. Stir a third of the egg whites into the melted chocolate mixture with a large metal spoon to loosen, then fold in the rest.

Divide the mixture between 6 dessert dishes or coffee cups. Cover them with cling film and chill for at least 1 hour. When you're ready to eat, take the dishes out of the fridge and uncover them. Tumble a few raspberries into the centre of each one, dust with sifted icing sugar and grate the remaining chocolate over the top. Serve this on the day of making.

Please note: this recipe contains raw egg whites.

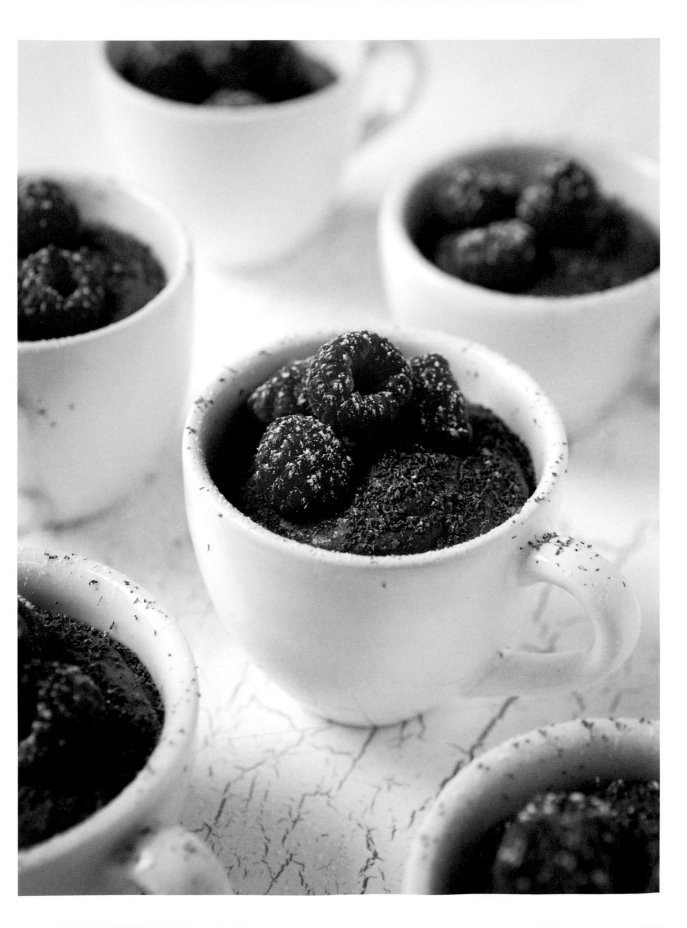

APPLE AND BLACKBERRY CORNFLAKE CRUMBLE

192 calories per portion

This contains far less fat than a traditional apple and blackberry crumble, thanks to our special topping. Cornflakes add lots of crunch but not too many calories.

Serves 6
Prep: 20 minutes
Cooking time: 30 minutes

75g caster sugar
½ tsp ground cinnamon
finely grated zest of ½ lemon
1 tbsp cornflour
450g Bramley cooking apples
  (about 2 medium apples)
300g fresh blackberries
25g fridge-cold butter, cut
  into cubes
25g plain flour
100g cornflakes

Preheat the oven to 200°C/Fan 180°C/Gas 6. Mix the sugar, cinnamon, lemon zest and cornflour in a large bowl. Peel, quarter and core the apples, then cut them into rough 1.5cm chunks and add them to the spiced sugar. Add the blackberries and toss everything well together.

Tip the apple and blackberry filling into a 1.5 litre pie dish or divide it between individual ramekins. Make sure you scrape all the sugary juices on top of the fruit too.

Put the butter, flour and cornflakes in a bowl and rub together between your fingertips until the mixture resembles coarse breadcrumbs. This should only take 2–3 minutes. Scatter the cornflake mixture evenly over the filling.

Bake in the centre of the oven for 30 minutes or until the crumble filling is bubbling, the fruit is tender and the topping is golden brown. Serve with low-fat custard or half-fat crème fraiche if you like, but don't forget that these add extra calories so watch it!

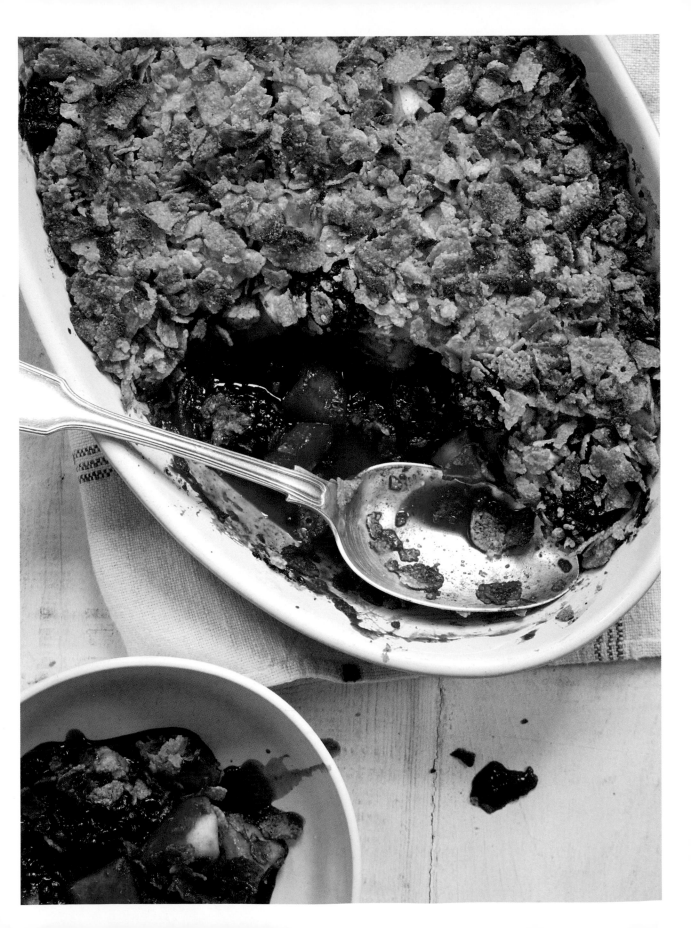

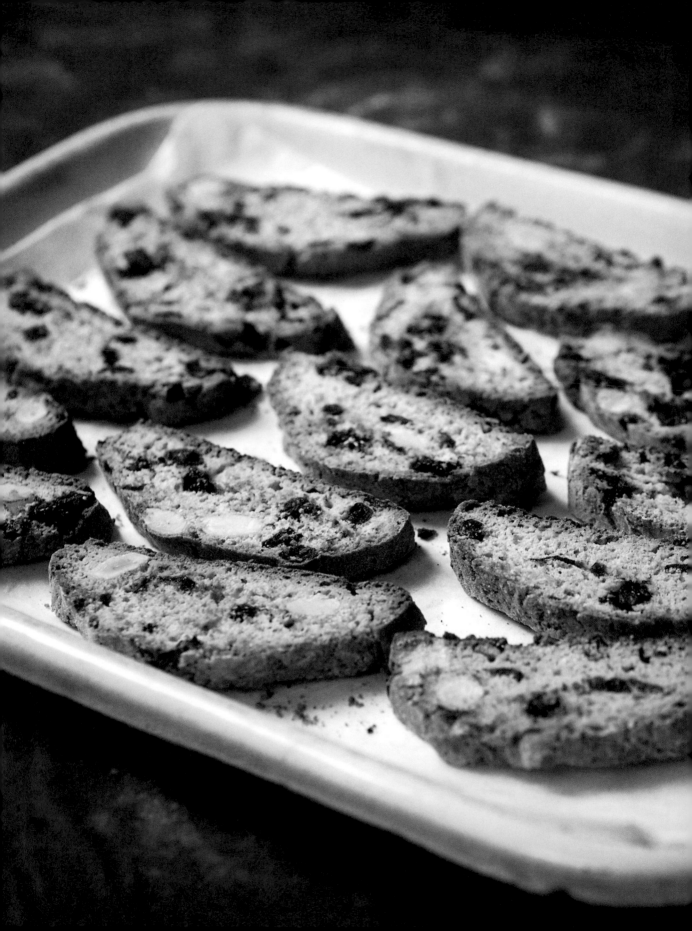

CHOCOLATE, ORANGE AND CRANBERRY BISCOTTI

53 calories per biscuit

Crunchy and tasty, these little biscotti are just the thing to serve with a coffee when you're in need of a hit of something sweet but don't want to overdo it. If you like, you can use orange-flavoured chocolate instead of the orange zest.

Preheat the oven to 180°C/Fan 160°C/Gas 4. Put the flour in a large bowl and stir in the baking powder, sugar and orange zest. Chop the chocolate into small pieces and put them in a colander. Shake them about a bit to get rid of any tiny pieces of chocolate, then tip the rest into the bowl with the flour.

Stir in the almonds and cranberries. Beat the whole egg and egg white with the vanilla extract and pour on to the flour. Mix with a wooden spoon and then your hands until the ingredients come together and form a stiff but pliable dough.

Put the dough on a well-floured board and roll it into a fat sausage-shape that's about 25cm long. Transfer this to a large baking tray lined with baking parchment and then flatten it slightly until it is about 2cm high.

Bake for 25–30 minutes until the dough is risen and firm but still looks fairly pale, then remove it from the oven and leave to cool on the baking tray for 10 minutes. Turn the oven down to 140°C/Fan 120°C/Gas 1. Put the cooked dough on a board and cut it into slices of about 1cm with a bread knife.

Put the biscuits back on the tray and bake them for another 25 minutes or until very lightly browned. They will crispen up as they dry. Leave the biscotti to cool, then store in an airtight container for up to 2 weeks.

Makes 30
Prep: 10 minutes, plus cooling
Cooking time: 35 minutes

175g plain flour, plus extra
  for dusting
1 tsp baking powder
100g caster sugar
finely grated zest of 1 medium
  orange
40g plain dark chocolate (about
  70% cocoa solids)
25g blanched almonds
40g dried cranberries
1 large egg, plus 1 large egg white
½ tsp vanilla extract

ALONG
SIDES

"All our recipes are calorie counted but sometimes we suggest that you might like to add a dollop of mash or a little rice alongside. We thought you might like to have some of our ways of preparing these, with calorie counts, so you know exactly what you are eating. These side dishes are also a useful way of bulking out a meal for non-dieting members of the family – they can have a big helping, you have a small one and there are smiles all round. We are also sharing our list of 100 calorie snacks for those awkward moments. The thing is – a biscuit eaten standing up in the kitchen is still a biscuit and it has calories so don't fool yourself that it doesn't count!"

Si

ROCKING RICE

We love our rice, but unfortunately in the past we've loved it too much for our own good. We used to help ourselves to huge piles of the lovely stuff and guess what? Rice has calories. Take good note of the quantities suggested here and you'll be fine.

Serves 4–6
Prep: 5 minutes
Cooking time: 10–12 minutes

about 1 litre cold water
175g easy-cook long-grain rice, such as Uncle Ben's

PLAIN RICE

168 calories per portion (if serving 4)
112 calories per portion (if serving 6)

Half fill a medium saucepan with the water and bring it to the boil. Stir the rice into the pan and bring the water back to the boil. Cook for 10–12 minutes, stirring occasionally, until the rice is tender. Drain the rice in a sieve and fluff it up with a fork before serving.

Serves 4–6
Prep: 10 minutes
Cooking time: 25 minutes

oil, for spraying
1 small onion, finely chopped
1 small garlic clove, crushed
½ tsp coriander seeds, lightly crushed
3 cardamom pods, lightly crushed
½ tsp cumin seeds
½ tsp fennel seeds
½ cinnamon stick
½ tsp ground turmeric
½ tsp black mustard seeds
1 bay leaf
175g basmati rice, rinsed in a sieve and drained
300ml chicken stock, made with 1 stock cube
freshly ground black pepper

PILAU RICE

170 calories per portion (if serving 4)
113 calories per portion (if serving 6)

Mist a medium non-stick sauté pan or lidded saucepan with oil and fry the onion and garlic over a medium heat for 3 minutes until very lightly browned, stirring frequently. Don't let the garlic burn or it will give your rice a bitter flavour.

Mix all the spices together and stir them into the pan. Add the bay leaf and cook for 2 minutes, stirring well. Stir the rice into the pan, then pour in the stock and season with freshly ground black pepper.

Bring to the boil and stir, then cover the pan with a tightly fitting lid. Turn the heat down and simmer the rice very gently for 15 minutes, then take the pan off the heat and leave to stand for 5 minutes. The rice should continue cooking without breaking up.

Remove the lid and fluff up the rice with a fork. If your rice isn't quite tender, add a little water, cover and cook for a few minutes more. Warn the family about the whole spices when you serve up!

MIXED VEGETABLE RICE

197 calories per portion (if serving 4)
131 calories per portion (if serving 6)

Serves 4–6
Prep: 10 minutes
Cooking time: 18 minutes

about 1 litre cold water
175g easy-cook long-grain rice, such as Uncle Ben's
oil, for spraying
1 small onion, finely chopped
1 red pepper, deseeded and cut into 1cm dice
50g frozen peas
flaked sea salt
freshly ground black pepper

Half fill a medium saucepan with the water and bring it to the boil. Stir the rice into the pan and bring it back to the boil. Cook for 10–12 minutes, stirring occasionally until tender.

Five minutes before the end of the cooking time, mist a medium non-stick saucepan with oil and place it over a low heat. Add the onion, and pepper and cook for 4 minutes, stirring regularly. Add the peas and cook for 1–2 minutes more, stirring. Drain the rice in a sieve and add it to the pan with the vegetables. Stir until well combined, season to taste with salt and pepper and serve.

MUSHROOM RICE

184 calories per portion (if serving 4)
123 calories per portion (if serving 6)

Serves 4–6
Prep: 10 minutes
Cooking time: 25 minutes

100g small chestnut button mushrooms, wiped
oil, for spraying
1 small onion, finely chopped
1 garlic clove, crushed
175g easy-cook long grain rice, such as Uncle Ben's
300ml chicken or vegetable stock, made with 1 stock cube
flaked sea salt
freshly ground black pepper

Thinly slice the mushrooms, cutting any larger ones in half before slicing. Mist a medium non-stick sauté pan or lidded saucepan with the oil and fry the onion and mushrooms over a medium heat for 3–4 minutes until lightly browned, stirring frequently.

Add the garlic and cook for a few seconds more, stirring constantly. Don't let the garlic burn or it will give your rice a bitter flavour. Stir the rice into the pan and pour in the stock. Season with a good pinch of salt and some freshly ground black pepper.

Bring to the boil and stir, then add a tightly fitting lid. Turn the heat down and simmer very gently for 15 minutes. Take the pan off the heat and leave to stand for 5 minutes. The rice should continue cooking without breaking up.

Remove the lid and fluff up the rice with a fork. If your rice isn't quite tender, add a little water, cover and cook for a few minutes more.

MARVELLOUS MASH

We can't do without our mash and here are some delicious ways to serve it without overdoing the calories. The portions are quite small, but they're enough to satisfy your carb cravings, while keeping to your diet. Be sure to serve lots of lovely veg alongside your main meal too.

CREAMY MASH

112 calories per portion

Serves 4
Prep: 6–8 minutes
Cooking time: 10–15 minutes

500g floury potatoes, preferably
   Maris Pipers or King Edwards
3 tbsp half-fat crème fraiche
flaked sea salt
freshly ground black pepper

Peel the potatoes and cut into them into chunks of about 3cm. Put them in a large saucepan, cover with cold water and bring to the boil. Cook for 10–15 minutes or until very tender – test with the tip of a knife. Drain the potatoes in a large colander and tip them back into the saucepan. Mash the cooked potatoes with the crème fraiche until smooth and season to taste.

CHAMP

132 calories per portion

Serves 4
Prep: 10 minutes
Cooking time: 10–15 minutes

500g floury potatoes, preferably
   Maris Pipers or King Edwards
15g butter
8 spring onions, trimmed and
   finely sliced
1 tbsp half-fat crème fraiche
flaked sea salt
freshly ground black pepper

Peel the potatoes and cut them into chunks of about 3cm. Put them in a large saucepan, cover with cold water and bring to the boil. Cook for 10–15 minutes or until the potatoes are very tender – test them with the tip of a knife. Meanwhile, melt the butter in a medium non-stick frying pan and cook the sliced spring onions for 1–2 minutes until softened, stirring constantly.

Drain the potatoes in a large colander and tip them into the pan with the spring onions. Add the crème fraiche, season with salt and lots of ground black pepper and mash roughly together.

500g floury potatoes, preferably
    Maris Pipers or King Edwards
1 tbsp half-fat crème fraiche
3 tbsp semi-skimmed milk
1 tbsp wholegrain mustard
flaked sea salt
freshly ground black pepper

500g floury potatoes, preferably
    Maris Pipers or King Edwards
½ tsp sunflower oil
2 rashers of rindless lean smoked
    streaky bacon, cut into 2cm pieces
½ medium onion, peeled and finely
    chopped
½ medium Savoy cabbage
    (about 300g)
3 tbsp semi-skimmed milk
flaked sea salt
freshly ground black pepper

MUSTARD MASH

110 calories per portion

Peel the potatoes and cut them into chunks of about 3cm. Put them in a large saucepan, cover with cold water and bring to the boil. Cook for 10–15 minutes or until the potatoes are very tender – test with the tip of a knife. Drain the potatoes in a large colander and tip them back into the saucepan. Mash with the crème fraiche and milk until smooth, then beat in the mustard and season to taste.

LOWER-CAL COLCANNON

157 calories per portion

Peel the potatoes and cut them into chunks of about 3cm. Put them in a large saucepan, cover with cold water and bring to the boil. Cook for 10–15 minutes or until very tender.

While the potatoes are cooking, brush the oil over the inside of a large non-stick frying pan and fry the bacon and onion together over a medium-high heat for 4–5 minutes or until the onion is softened and the bacon is lightly browned, stirring regularly.

Remove any damaged leaves from the cabbage and cut it in half. Cut out the tough central core and thinly shred the leaves. Add the shredded cabbage to the pan with the bacon and onion and cook for 6–8 minutes until softened, stirring regularly. Add a tablespoon of water to the pan every couple of minutes to prevent the cabbage burning. Remove from the heat.

Drain the potatoes in a large colander and tip them back into the saucepan. Mash with the milk until smooth and season to taste. Tip the potatoes into the same pan as the softened cabbage and stir together over a low heat until hot and well combined. Transfer to a warmed dish and serve.

JAUNTY JACKET POTATOES

169 calories per 225g potato

Jacket potatoes make a great easy meal and here are some of our favourite ways of dressing them up. If you're in a rush you can microwave your potatoes if you like, but we like them best piping hot and crunchy skinned straight from the oven.

Serves 4
Prep: 1–2 minutes
Cooking time: 1 hour

4 medium potatoes
   (about 225g each)
flaked sea salt
freshly ground black pepper

Preheat the oven to 220°C/Fan 200°C/Gas 7. Prick the potatoes a few times with a fork – this should stop the skins splitting.

Carefully place the potatoes directly on to the oven shelf – watch out, it will be very hot. Bake for 1 hour or until crisp on the outside and soft and fluffy inside. Baking the potatoes directly on the oven shelf helps them to crisp all over.

Remove the potatoes from the oven – be careful, they will be hot! Make a deep cross in the centre of each potato with a sharp knife and open it out a bit so it can hold the filling. Season with salt and pepper or fill with your favourite of our delicious fillings.

Serves 4
Prep: 10 minutes
Cooking time: 10 minutes

2 large eggs, fridge cold
100g green beans, trimmed and cut
   into 3cm lengths
2 x 130g cans of tuna steak in water,
   drained
12 cherry tomatoes, quartered
75g pitted green olives in brine,
   drained and halved
1 tbsp low-calorie dressing
flaked sea salt
freshly ground black pepper

TUNA NIÇOISE FILLING

266 calories per portion with potato

Half fill a small saucepan with cold water and bring to the boil. Add the eggs, bring the water back to the boil and simmer for 9 minutes. While the eggs are cooking, put another small pan of water on to boil. Add the green beans, bring back to the boil and simmer for 2 minutes. Drain in a colander and run under cold water until cool.

Carefully remove the eggs with a slotted spoon and place them under cold running water until cool, then peel and cut into quarters. Put the tuna in a large mixing bowl and toss with the green beans, cherry tomatoes and olives. Drizzle with the dressing and season with salt and pepper. Spoon the tuna into the jacket potatoes and pop the egg quarters on top to serve.

Serves 4
Prep: 5 minutes
Cooking time: 3 minutes

415g can of baked beans
4 reduced-fat cheese triangles, halved
4 spring onions, trimmed and finely sliced
flaked sea salt
freshly ground black pepper

CHEESY BEANS FILLING

280 calories per portion with potato

Heat the beans in a saucepan until hot, stirring. Divide them between the hot potatoes and top with cheese triangles. Scatter over the spring onions and season with salt and black pepper. If you don't fancy the beans, serve the potatoes, cheese and spring onions with a colourful mixed salad instead. You'll save yourself some calories too.

Serves 4
Prep: 10 minutes

¼ small white cabbage
1 medium carrot, peeled
5 spring onions, trimmed
75g light mayonnaise
175g fat-free natural yoghurt
flaked sea salt
freshly ground black pepper

CREAMY COLESLAW FILLING

266 calories per portion with potato

Put the cabbage on a board and cut out the central core. Shred the cabbage as finely as you can and put it all in a bowl. Coarsely grate the carrot, slice the spring onions finely and add them to the cabbage. Spoon the mayonnaise and yoghurt over the vegetables and mix until thoroughly combined. Season with a good pinch of salt and plenty of black pepper, then divide the filling between the hot potatoes.

Serves 4
Prep: 10 minutes

---

2 tbsp light mayonnaise
4 tbsp fat-free natural yoghurt
2 tsp tomato ketchup
100g cooked peeled prawns, thawed if frozen
1 baby gem lettuce
12 cherry tomatoes, quartered
50g cucumber, quartered lengthways and sliced
pinch of paprika, to garnish (optional)
lemon wedges, for serving
freshly ground black pepper

PRAWN COCKTAIL FILLING

233 calories per portion with potato

Mix the mayonnaise, yoghurt and tomato ketchup in a small bowl until well combined. Drain the prawns and stir them into the sauce, then season with black pepper.

Separate and rinse the lettuce leaves and toss them with the tomatoes and cucumber. Divide the salad between the hot jacket potatoes and top with the prawns. Sprinkle with the paprika, if using and serve with lemon wedges to squeeze on top.

PERFECT PASTA

Huge pasta dishes will make you pile on the pounds quickly, so get used to smaller serving sizes and bulk up with fresh vegetables instead. Serve these pasta dishes with a lovely mixed salad if you like.

BROCCOLI PASTA

345 calories per portion

Serves 2
Prep: 5 minutes
Cooking time: 12 minutes

75g dried pasta shapes, such as fusilli or penne
300g broccoli, cut into small florets
25g pine nuts, preferably Italian
2 tbsp fresh basil pesto sauce
flaked sea salt
freshly ground black pepper

Half fill a large saucepan with cold water and bring it to the boil. Add the pasta, stir well and return to the boil. Cook for 8 minutes, stirring occasionally. Add the broccoli to the pan, bring the water back to the boil and cook for another 2–3 minutes until both the broccoli and the pasta are tender.

While the pasta and broccoli are cooking, toast the pine nuts in a small frying pan over a medium heat until they're lightly browned, stirring regularly.

Drain the pasta and broccoli in a colander, then tip them back into the saucepan. Sprinkle with the pine nuts and stir in the pesto sauce Season with a good pinch of salt and lots of ground black pepper

PRAWN PASTA SALAD

304 calories per portion

Serves 2
Prep: 10 minutes
Cooking time: about 10 minutes

75g dried pasta shapes, such as fusilli or penne
3 tbsp light mayonnaise
1 tbsp cold water
2 tsp tomato ketchup
150g cooked, peeled prawns, thawed if frozen and drained
10 cherry tomatoes, halved
¼ cucumber, cut into 1.5cm dice
1 medium carrot, coarsely grated
4–5 romaine lettuce leaves, shredded, to serve
freshly ground black pepper

Half fill a large saucepan with cold water and bring it to the boil. Add the pasta, stir well and return to the boil. Cook for 8–10 minutes, or until tender, stirring occasionally. Rinse the pasta in a colander under running water until cold. Drain it well in a colander.

Put the mayonnaise and water in a large bowl and stir until smooth. Add the tomato ketchup and mix thoroughly, then add the pasta to the bowl and toss lightly.

Scatter the prawns, tomatoes, cucumber and grated carrot on top. Season with a few twists of ground black pepper and gently toss all the ingredients together. Serve on top of shredded romaine lettuce leaves if you like. Just right for lunchboxes and picnics.

TAGLIATELLE CARBONARA

279 calories per portion

Serves 2
Prep: 10 minutes
Cooking time: 10–12 minutes

75g dried tagliatelle pasta
2 rashers of rindless lean smoked
    back bacon
oil, for spraying
200g small chestnut mushrooms,
    sliced
1 medium courgette, trimmed
    and cut into 1.5cm dice
10 cherry tomatoes, halved
4 tbsp half-fat crème fraiche
15g finely grated Parmesan cheese
freshly ground black pepper

Half fill a large saucepan with cold water and bring it to the boil. Add the pasta, stir well and return to the boil. Cook for 10–12 minutes or until tender, stirring occasionally. While the pasta is cooking, trim any visible fat off the bacon and cut the rashers into 2cm-wide strips. Mist a medium non-stick frying pan with oil and fry the bacon and mushrooms together for 4 minutes over a medium-high heat until they're starting to brown, stirring regularly.

Add the courgette and cook for 2 minutes, then add the tomatoes and cook for 1 minute more. Drain the pasta in a colander, then tip it back into the saucepan. Add the bacon, mushrooms, courgette and tomatoes. Spoon over the crème fraiche and add the cheese and a few twists of ground black pepper. Toss lightly together.

SPICY BACON AND TOMATO PASTA

302 calories per portion

Serves 2
Prep: 10 minutes
Cooking time: 10–12 minutes

75g dried pasta shapes, such
    as penne
2 rashers of rindless lean smoked
    back bacon
oil, for spraying
1 large yellow pepper, deseeded
    and cut into 2.5cm chunks
125g tenderstem broccoli, trimmed
    and cut into 2cm diagonal slices
150ml cold water
150g tomato and basil sauce, fresh
    or from a jar (look for one with
    no more than 6g fat per 100g)
2 tbsp half-fat crème fraiche
heaped ½ tsp dried chilli flakes
freshly ground black pepper

Half fill a large saucepan with cold water and bring it to the boil. Add the pasta, stir well and return to the boil. Cook for 10–12 minutes or until tender, stirring occasionally. While the pasta is cooking, trim any visible fat off the bacon and cut the rashers into 2cm wide strips. Mist a medium non-stick frying pan with oil and fry the bacon for 1½–2 minutes over a medium heat until lightly browned, stirring regularly. Tip it on to a plate and return the pan to the heat.

Add the pepper and stir-fry for 2 minutes until lightly browned, then add the broccoli and stir-fry for a minute with the pepper. Pour the water into the pan and simmer the vegetables for 4 minutes, stirring regularly. Add a little extra water if it completely evaporates before the end of the cooking time.

Stir in the cooked bacon, pasta sauce, crème fraiche and chilli flakes and cook until the sauce is hot, stirring constantly. Drain the pasta in a colander then tip it back into the saucepan. Add the hot bacon sauce, toss together, then season with black pepper and serve.

WHAT YOU GET FOR 100 CALORIES

When you're dieting, there are times when you need a little extra something. Perhaps a side dish of rice or some potatoes, a smidgen of cheese or a not too naughty snack. Here's a list of things that we like to have once in a while and they all contain about 100 calories, give or take a few, so won't break your calorie budget. That does mean sticking to the portions we've listed though, no more, and we mean that. Be sure to measure and weigh whatever you're going to have and avoid the temptation to take that extra handful. Remember – twice the portion means twice the calories!

WHEAT, RICE, POTATOES AND RYE

½ white or wholemeal pitta bread

1 slice of white, brown or wholemeal bread

1 crumpet

1 small bread roll

½ plain bagel

½ English muffin

2 small plain oatcakes

5 plain breadsticks

3 rye crispbreads

2½ rice or corn cakes

1 heaped palmful (25g) uncooked pasta shapes

1 small portion cooked pasta shapes (75g) about half a mugful

1 small palmful uncooked rice (30g)

1 small portion cooked rice (75g)

1 small palmful uncooked couscous (30g)

1 small baked potato

3 small new potatoes

1 medium roast potato (65g)

30g dry egg or rice noodles

2 ready-made frozen Yorkshire puddings

1 small flour or corn tortilla wrap

DAIRY

25g piece of hard cheese, such as cheddar

30g wedge of French cheese, such as Brie

30g slice of soft goat's cheese

40g feta cheese

2 heaped tsp butter, vegetable or olive oil spread

1 ½ tbsp double cream

4 tbsp half-fat crème fraiche

2 tbsp full-fat soft cheese

1 small low-fat fruit yoghurt

200ml semi-skimmed milk

200ml 0% fat Greek yoghurt

100ml cottage cheese

5 small mozzarella pearls

ALCOHOL

1 small (125ml) glass of white, red or rosé wine

2 x single gin or vodka with low-calorie tonic

2 x single rum and diet cola

125ml glass champagne

½ pt (284ml) glass lager or bitter

OILS AND DRESSINGS

1 tbsp olive, sunflower or vegetable oil

1 tbsp mayonnaise

2 tbsp light mayonnaise

2 tbsp salad cream

SAVOURY SNACKS

1 large hard-boiled egg

½ small avocado

20g prawn crackers

2 poppadoms

100g olives, in brine

125g baked beans

50g sundried tomatoes, in oil, drained well

24g pack of Twiglets/Quavers

3 tbsp houmous

20g unsalted peanuts

MEAT AND FISH

3 slices of Parma ham

75g cooked ham

75g roasted chicken or turkey breast

100g canned tuna in spring water or brine

50g corned beef

75g smoked salmon

1 half-fat pork sausage

50g hot-smoked salmon

FRUIT AND NUTS

150g blueberries

1 medium banana

200g fresh pineapple chunks

1 large pear

2 small nectarines

150g bunch of grapes

75g ready-to-eat prunes

40g raisins

250ml unsweetened apple juice

2 large plums

40g mixed dried fruit

2 slices of watermelon

10 ready-to-eat apricots

15 blanched almonds

12 unsalted cashew nuts

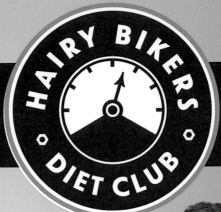

HAIRY BIKERS
DIET CLUB

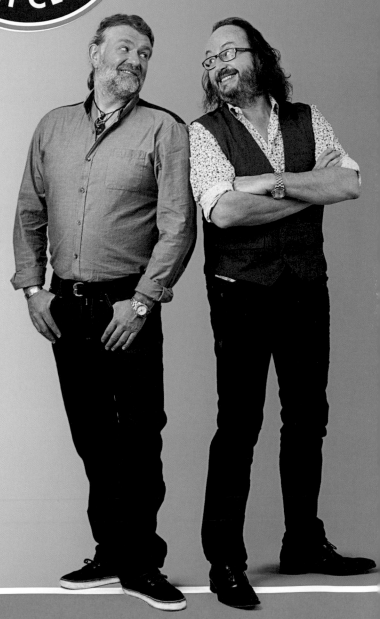

From the very start of their calorie-counting journey to today's ongoing mission to keep those pounds and inches at bay, Si and Dave continue to share their inspiring weight-loss discoveries.

And now it's your turn!

The Hairy Bikers' Diet Club is your chance to join forces with like-minded food lovers in a Hairy Bikers' community designed to inspire and motivate you on a monthly basis. So whether you're proud of your achievements or need a friendly nudge in the right direction, now's the time to get involved.

Sign up to The Hairy Bikers' Diet Club today to share your dieting goals and experiences with fellow members and feast your eyes on exclusive news, recipes and extra bite-sized morsels of dieting goodness.

FIND OUT MORE AT
WWW.HAIRYBIKERS.COM/CLUB

INDEX

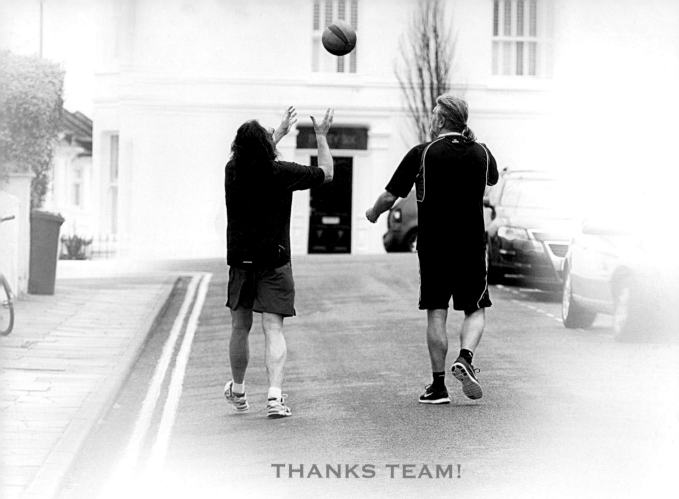

THANKS TEAM!

Yet again, Team Hairy has helped us put together a really fantastic book. We'd like to say a huge thank you to everyone for all your hard work.

Big thanks to diet expert Justine Pattison, who worked with us on the recipes and shared her encyclopedic nutritional knowledge and advice. And we'd like to thank her tireless team of recipe testers: Lauren Brignell, Kirsty Thomas, Angela Platt, Gileng Salter and Jane Gwillim, as well as the valiant kitchen helpers and washers-up, Jess and Emily PB.

Andrew Hayes-Watkins is an amazing photographer and the photos he's taken for this book are just superb – we love them. Many, many thanks too to Lisa Harrison and Anna Burges-Lumsden for preparing all the food so beautifully for the pictures, and to Loulou Clark for finding all the great props. Thanks to Loulou and to Lucie Stericker for all their work on the design – they are both works of art themselves and they've certainly made our book something special. And thank you to Jinny Johnson for making sense of our garbled ramblings, and to the wonderful Amanda Harris for steering the whole ship with such skill.

Last but not least, a very special thank you to all at James Grant Management, who look after us so brilliantly. Nicola Ibison put us on the right track with the Hairy Dieters project from the word go, so massive thanks to Nicola and to Natalie Zietcer, Tessa Findlay, Rowan Lawton and Eugenie Furniss – you're superstars and we love you all.

We'd also like to thank the Optomen team who worked so hard on the original Hairy Dieters television series.